The Flower Remedy Book

THE FLOWER REMEDY BOOK

A COMPREHENSIVE GUIDE TO OVER 700 FLOWER ESSENCES

Jeffrey Garson Shapiro, H.D., Ph.D.

North Atlantic Books
Berkeley, California

Published by
North Atlantic Books
P.O. Box 12327
Berkeley, California 94712

Cover digital art based on a drawing by Harry Robins
Cover and book design by Legacy Media
Printed in the United States of America

The Flower Remedy Book is sponsored by the Society for the Study of Native Arts and Sciences, a nonprofit educational corporation whose goals are to develop an educational and crosscultural perspective linking various scientific, social, and artistic fields; to nurture a holistic view of arts, sciences, humanities, and healing; and to publish and distribute literature on the relationship of mind, body, and nature.

Library of Congress Cataloging-in-Publication Data

Shapiro, Jeffrey G.
    The flower remedy book : a comprehensive guide to over
700 flower essences / Jeffrey G. Shapiro
    p. cm.
    ISBN 1-55643-296-8 (alk. paper)
1. Flowers—Therapeutic use. 2. Homeopathy—Materia
medica and therapeutics. I. Title.
RX615.F55S45 1999
615'.321—DC21   98-39493
                                          CIP

1 2 3 4 5 6 7 8 9 / 03 02 01 00 99

*This book is dedicated
to my first born, Jeremy,
born July 6, 1998.*

The love I couldn't wait to meet.

Acknowledgments

I would like to gratefully acknowledge the following individuals:

John Zulli, Marlan Goodwin, and everyone else at Curentur University for giving me the opportunity to explore, learn, and love homeopathy and flower essences;

Al Hoagland, Jr. and Victoria Easterbrook for being there in the beginning;

Lila Devi and Yolanda LaCombe for sharing their wisdom about flower essences;

Dana Ullman, a man I have long respected from a distance, who now has given me the opportunity to publish this work;

To Linda and Herb Krakower, Michael and Susan Garson, Melissa, Heather and Matt, and the rest of my family for being a part of my life;

To my mentor and friend, Jeanne Zeeb.

And to my wife, Jennifer,the absolute love of my life.

Table of Contents

Foreword

I recently stumbled upon this scribbled message on a piece of paper tacked between notices of healing services on a posterboard in a holistic health center. Entitled *A Short History of Medicine*, it offers a cure for the simple earache.

2000 BC: Here, eat this root.
1000 AD: That root is heathen. Here, say this prayer.
1850 AD: That prayer is superstition. Here, drink this potion.
1940 AD: That potion is snake oil. Here, swallow this pill.
1985 AD: That pill is ineffective. Here, take this antibiotic.
2000 AD: That antibiotic is artificial. Here, eat this root.

One is tempted to add a final entry, possibly 2001 AD, if not earlier: "That root is good. But to get to the root of the problem: here, try this flower essence." In this century, flower essences have shown themselves to be an important step forward in natural medicine. Many essence lines available today are backed by extensive case studies and direct testimonials, confirming their efficacy many times over. Although the definitions of *how* they actually work are many and varied, the plain fact is that they *do* work: for people, pets, and plants. And they work simply, painlessly and inexpensively. In harmony with nature, these remedies vibrationally coax us to live likewise.

Flower essences balance our otherwise chaotic, stress-ridden lives. Somewhat like tapping us on the shoulder, they softly say, "Remember what a walk in the woods feels like, or digging your toes into the cold wet sand of the seashore?" In describing how essences work, the credited father of flower remedies, Dr. Edward Bach, waxed poetic with similes and metaphors rather than clinical descriptions. They work, he reflected, much like watching a beautiful sunset or listening to uplifting music.

All properly and hygienically prepared flower essences do the same thing: they return us to a state of balance. Once they prime the pump of our own life force, so to speak, we can then heal ourselves — or at least make significant progress in that direction. Flower essences give us the key so that we can open the door. Which is much easier, isn't it, than trying to get in through the window?

To continue the metaphor, *The Flower Remedy Book: A Comprehensive Guide to Over 700 Flower Essences* provides us with a key ring of many such keys. Numerous essence lines — of which nine companies are presented here, my own included — offer a seemingly infinite variety of flower essences. Dr. Garson Shapiro's book is also a repertory of my friends: the developers of the various essences whom I have met (with the exception of Green Hope Farm and Pegasus).

As indeed the fruit falls not far from the tree, the developers themselves, in almost uncanny ways, resemble their essence lines: gentle, approachable, beautiful in spirit, and profoundly committed to helping humanity heal itself. It seems that we flower essence developers have all come to earth at this particular time, a smaller family within a greater one, to expand this extraordinary healing science and art.

I met Richard Katz, of the esteemed Flower Essence Services, in the early eighties. How coincidental that our companies both originated and reside in California's Sierra Nevada Foothills! At that time, we made several essences together. I was to meet his wife and partner, Patricia Kaminski, some years later. In Richard, I sensed a level-headed visionary who, along with Patricia, has brought integrity and credibility to the flower essence world. This sense of instant recognition and kinship has accompanied my meeting with practically every other flower essence developer since that time.

Julian Barnard, of the English Healing Herbs, and I met in a most comical way: in our bathrobes in the tiny kitchen of our shared bungalow accommodations for Findhorn's groundbreaking '97 International Flower Essence Conference in Scotland. "I've heard so much about you," we said almost simultaneously, a bit embarrassed by the impromptu nature of the circumstances. A gentle man who radiates clarity, compassion, and sincerity, Julian has done much to further the message of the flowers.

Australia, a land of rich mystery, may rightfully boast two strong flower essence companies: Ian White's Australian Bush Essences and Vasudeva and Kadambii Barneo's Australian Living Essences. Ian's generation-to-generation background in communing with herbs and flowers spills over in the magnetic enthusiasm of his essence presentation. Vasudeva (I wasn't able to meet his wife, then weeks away from her due date), as gentle-spirited as the flowers themselves, weaves an aboriginal spell with well-narrated slides and the devotion of his work.

Steve Johnson of the Alaskan Flower Essence Project, quiet and gentle, reflects the stillness of the Alaskan landscape which he honors through his essence line. And Machaelle Small Wright brings one to a front row seat at the Perelandra gardens through her down-home, thoroughly affable presentation of her essence line.

Dr. Garson Shapiro — or Jeffrey, as I call him — is to be commended for this labor-of-love repertory: a resource guide that makes flower essences easier to work with, more accessible, and better known. Himself a Grape theme according to the framework of my essence line, love and compassion are the guiding motives of his work. (Replacing the archaic and somewhat condemning "type remedy" concept which defines an individual according to predominant negative personality traits, the theme essence construct elevates one by identification with major positive qualities: thus the loving, embracing quality of the Grape theme.) In the time I've known Jeffrey, I have found in him a humanitarian and a healer, and one committed to the truth of nature and the nature of truth.

In discovering this book, you have found a practical and resourceful gem. I hope you use it well, and lovingly, as it was compiled.

Lila Devi
Founder of Master's Flower Essences
Nevada City, California
April, 1998

Introduction

This book started out as a very personal project. During my course of studies in homeopathy, I discovered and fell in love with flower essences. I found them to be a wonderful healing art in their own right, as well as a marvelous complement to homeopathy. As I explored flower essences my "collection" of remedies continued to grow. Soon I found that I had literally hundreds of essences from around the world from a full variety of manufacturers. As I would try to determine which essence or essences were most appropriate for the particular case at hand, I had to juggle nine or so different books at a time. Each maker of essences put out their own guide to cover the particular remedies they made. There existed no one source which was comprehensive, accurate, and easy to use.

At this point I decided that I should undertake a project of developing a comprehensive guide for myself. In homeopathy, this type of guide is called a repertory. It lists individual symptoms with the indicated remedies for that symptom (this is called a rubric). This was the model I chose to follow. The introduction of the repertory revolutionized the practice of homeopathy because it allowed practitioners to go beyond their existing knowledge and experience with certain remedies. I figured, that at very least, the introduction of a comprehensive repertory of flower essences would revolutionize my ability to utilize these remedies.

To start constructing this work, I first had to identify the flower essences to be included. Each of the makers of flower remedies has their own roster of essences, some overlap with other makers, but many do not. I realized that the only way to compile the repertory was to identify the makers of the essences. I started to survey retail outlets and various practitioners of flower essence therapy. From this, I was able to determine the nine most readily available lines of essences. This would include some 700 or so essences.

The next step was to identify the symptoms that would make up the rubrics. To do this, I sat down with a homeopathic repertory, as well as with the various flower essence guides I could find. I selected all the rubrics that seemed appropriate and added a few I thought were missing.

This done, the rubrics needed to be built. I realized that it would be helpful to do two additional things to the rubrics, beyond just listing the names of the remedies. One was to annotate the essence, to give a brief description of how that flower remedy might help to address the symptom. The other was to identify the makers of that particular remedy. This, I thought, would make it much easier to then find the remedy and employ it. (Note that the repertory is divided into two sections, one for Mental/Emotional Symptoms, the other for Physical Symptoms. Only the Mental/Emotional Section includes the annotations. This is because flower essences have an effect on a person's mental/emotional state. Any physical effect is a result of the mental/emotional cause being balanced.)

Finally, the rubrics were built by reviewing the various guides to flower essences and matching the essences to the appropriate symptoms.

As I started to share the ideas for my repertory, I found that others were requesting a copy of the completed work. The rest is now history. I brought my manuscript to the attention of Dana Ullman. Through his interest, you now have the published version of my personal project.

One last note. As so often happens, after completing this work, a few other flower remedies and makers of flower remedies were brought to my attention. These may be appropriate for inclusion in a future revision.

Jeffrey Garson Shapiro
June, 1998

THE
FLOWER
REMEDY
BOOK

A Brief History and Overview of Flower Essences

Flower essences as a healing art was introduced in modern times by Dr. Edward Bach. Bach was born in 1886 near Birmingham, England. He was trained as a physician and spent a number of years as a bacteriologist, focusing on chronic disease. He started to become disenchanted with conventional medicine and the notion of alleviating symptoms of disease rather than their cause. He started to explore vaccine therapy and then was drawn to homeopathy and the principle of treating the whole person. A set of homeopathic remedies, called the Bach Nosodes (or Bowel Nosodes), prepared from various bacteria which are found in the human intestinal tract, is Bach's legacy to homeopathy.

Bach came to believe that emotional states were the cause of physical disease. He started to group different personality types which led to certain patterns of health imbalances. In 1930, Bach gave up his medical practice and spent the final six years of his life in the fields of rural England exploring various flowers and their effect on human emotions and health. Apparently a sensitive soul, he was drawn to certain plants and determined their therapeutic use by testing them on himself. Ultimately, the world was left with the thirty-eight healing flowers that make up the Bach Flower Remedies.

Bach himself offered no scientific explanation as to how flower essences worked. He did, however, leave hundreds of case histories detailing the positive effects of his flower remedies.

For many years, the Bach remedies remained a small and little known form of healing art. Then in the 1970s and 1980s, individuals started to discover or re-discover the work of Edward Bach. A number of people, independently, in various parts of the world, started to develop and expand the opus of flower essences. Lila Devi, founder and director of the Master's Flower Essences, incorporated the philosophy and teachings of Paramhansa Yogananda, an Indian yogi and teacher. From this, she developed the twenty garden essences made from fruit and vegetable blossoms which make up the Master's line. Not far from Lila Devi, Richard Katz and Patricia

Kaminski were pioneering and developing flower essences made from North American plants.

In Australia, Vasudeva Barnao and his wife, Kadambii, developed the Living Essences of Australia by incorporating the ancient tradition of flower essence therapy used by the Aboriginal Nyoongah people. Elsewhere in Australia, Ian White explored the flowers of the Australian Bush to develop the Australian Bush Essences.

Back in the United States, Steve Johnson was encouraged by the work of Katz and Kaminski and formed the Alaskan Flower Essence Project. In New Hampshire, Molly Sheehan has developed an eclectic mix of essences from New England, the Adirondack mountains, and the Island of Bermuda.

In the Blue Ridge Mountains of Virginia, Machaelle Small Wright established the Perelandra Garden, a nature research center. She developed rose and garden essences from the vegetables, herbs, roses, and other flowers which grow at Perelandra.

Today, flower essence use is growing rapidly. Once hard to find, various flower remedies are showing up for sale in markets, pharmacies, and other stores around the country. A full variety of health professionals incorporate flower essences into their practice, from MDs and psychiatrists, psychologists and other therapists, homeopaths and acupuncturists to massage therapists and even personal trainers.

How Flower Essences are Made

Traditionally, there are two formats for making essences, the Sun Method and the Boiling Method.

The Sun Method

In this method, a glass bowl is filled with water—Bach himself suggested the use of local spring water. The flowers or buds are then placed in the bowl and set out in the sun for a number of hours. The solarization traps the essence of the flower in the water. This liquid is then mixed with an equal part of preserving agent. Bach used brandy. Others use vodka, grain alcohol, vegetable glycerin, or red shiso and vinegar. This is called the mother tincture. The mother tincture can then be used to make stock bottles by placing a number of drops—different individuals use different numbers but 2–7 seems about average—in a dropper bottle filled with a mixture of water and preserving agent. This stock bottle is then stirred or "succussed"—shaking the bottle while impacting it in the palm of your hand, on a leather bound book or other similar surface. The purpose of this stirring or succussion is to invigorate, imprint, or spread the flower essence throughout the solution in the bottle.

The Boiling Method

Similar to the Sun Method, the Boiling Method uses a pot in which the flowers or buds are boiled in water and allowed to simmer. The boiling traps the essence of the flower in the water. After this water is allowed to cool and is filtered, the same process occurs to preserve the essence and to bottle it.

How Flower Essences Work

Bach himself offered no scientific explanation for how or why flower essences work. Still today, there is no explanation as to how and why they work. Pharmaceuticals, herbs, and nutritionals can all be explained because they work by causing chemical reactions in the body. Flower essences, like homeopathy and acupuncture, are energetic medicines. At least theoretically, what energy medicines do is act like a trigger for the body's own ability to heal. In the case of flower essences, the common belief is that the energetic pattern of the flower essence is similar to the energetic pattern of the individual's emotional state. The body responds to the stimulus of the flower essence and works to bring itself back into balance. This process tends to be very gentle and without side effects.

This can be illustrated using the following analogy (the room repre-sents the human body, the first tuning fork represents the flower remedy and the second, matching tuning fork represents the emotional state):

One enters a room holding a tuning fork. In this room, the walls are lined with many tuning forks, each one of a different musical note. If you strike the fork being held, it will start to vibrate. Nothing will happen to any of the other tuning forks in the room, except if there is one of the same note. It too will start to vibrate.

Although how flower essences work cannot be concretely proven, the clinical evidence of case histories from the last sixty-five plus years cer-tainly gives credence to their effectiveness. Today, many flower essence makers collect case histories and do their own clinical trials of testing reme-dies to document their effects. Flower Essence Services, in Nevada City, California has devoted an entire center for the purpose of testing flower remedies and collecting case histories from practitioners and users of flower essences.

Determining the Indications for Flower Essences

Edward Bach used his own intuition to initially identify a flower essence's purpose. Many of the flower essences being made today were first inspired by intuition, observation, conjecture, folklore, and even trance channeling. For the most part, regardless of the original inspiration for making an essence, most makers test them and collect clinical information. It should be pointed out that there are some makers who do not do this. One company, in particular, Pegasus Products, is controversial in flower essence circles because they rely almost exclusively on trance channeling to determine a flower's purpose. It is for you to determine whether or not this invalidates any or all of their essences. I can state that although I have not used all 700 or so of the remedies included in this book, I have personally witnessed and experienced positive results from essences from each of the flower essence manufacturers whose essences are included in this work.

Listed below is a brief summary of how each of the makers of essences included in this repertory make their determinations. This information is taken from the written and oral material from the makers themselves:

The Alaskan Flower Essence Project

Founder Steve Johnson was so moved by the wildflower paradise of Alaska that he started to test the Alaskan flowers that now make up this collection. He relies on intuition, his own experiences, devic and environmental guidance, and clinical reports from those who have taken or administered the Alaskan essences.

Australian Bush Flower Essences

Through meditation and spiritual guidance, founder Ian White initially determined the purpose of the flower essences that make up the Australian Bush line. Subsequent to this, observation of the clinical effects of the essences, kinesiology, Kirlian photography, and unconventional medical diagnostic equipment such as Vega and Morley machines are used to check the accuracy of his initial determinations.

Flower Essence Services

FES flowers are made and their effects documented at Terra Flora, a seventeen-acre, private research and educational center. FES has a formal research program open to those who wish to participate. FES invites people to submit clinical observations and case studies; controlled clinical studies; studies of subtle plant properties based on the principles of spiritual science; and research on detecting, analyzing, and interpreting the presence of subtle forces within flower essences.

Green Hope Farm

Founder Molly Sheehan has determined the indications for the Green Hope essences "in partnership with Nature, specifically the wonderful Angels and Elementals." Like Dr. Bach, she feels that she must go through a personal experience with each essence. If clinical experience reveals additional information about an essence, she returns to the garden to try to experience this new data herself.

Living Essences of Australia

Founders Vasudeva and Kadambii Barnao have determined the indications for the Living Essences through many years of testing and documenting the effects of their flower essences and by incorporating the ancient flower essence therapy tradition of the Australian Aboriginal Nyoongah peoples.

Master's Flower Essences

The twenty fruit and vegetable blossom essences that make up the Master's line were developed based on the initial interpretations of East Indian master teacher Paramhansa Yogananda. Acknowledging that foods heal us psychologically as well as nutritionally, this flower-food connection also provides valuable clues to essence assessment. These have since been extensively documented through collected case histories and testimonials—about people, pets, and plants—by founder and director Lila Devi and others whose practice employs the Master's Flower Essences.

Pegasus Products

"Pegasus Products are the result of prayer and spiritual guidance." The indicated uses for the Pegasus essences are primarily determined by trance channeling. The personal experiences of users of Pegasus essences are taken into consideration.

Perelandra

Perelandra is a nature research center. Its research focus is on creating a garden environment which is balanced so that everything in the environment enhances the life and health of all else in the garden. The Perelandra

Rose and Garden Essences are one result of the work being done at Perelandra. The indicated uses of the essences are derived from founder Machaelle Small Wright's "telepathic attunement with nature and the specific varieties of the plants involved, plus the results of research with the essences themselves."

What to Expect From Flower Essences

Flower essences tend to work quickly. Depending on the situation, the person, and depth of the issue, flower essences begin working in a matter of seconds, minutes or days. The effect of flower remedies may be very noticeable, as in the first two of the case studies below. Or they may be more subtle, with changes occurring over a period of time, as in the third case study. At times, others may notice the changes effected by the essences before you do.

Flower essences can have a long-term effect if they trigger the body to re-balance the emotional state that is out of balance. For issues where the cause of the imbalance remains, the effects may be shorter term, as in the case of being in an unhappy relationship or job situation.

Flower remedies work primarily on the mental/emotional plane. However, when physical situations arise as a result of an emotional imbalance, flower remedies have been known to be helpful in alleviating physical symptoms by triggering the body to correct the emotional cause.

Some Brief Personal Experiences

The power and effectiveness of flower essences will never cease to amaze me. The following four accounts are particularly dramatic:

Case Number One:

I was working with an adorable three-year-old boy. He was quite charming and loving. His problem was his lack of complete potty training. Although he did use the bathroom, he still had "accidents." These accidents upset him a great deal, and he started to tend toward constipation. His mother thought he had some type of emotional blockage to this rite of passage of being a big boy.

Considering this, I suggested that the boy be given tomato essence (Master's brand was used). Tomato essence is for the "purposeful warrior" to overcome "emotional blockages." The boy's mother gave him the remedy—and within a matter of seconds he defecated in his pants. This happened each of the four times he was given the tomato essence, until his mother stopped giving it to him—for obvious reasons. After this, the boy's toileting issues disappeared. He was also given the tomato essence at a later date, and the "accidents" did not recur.

Case Number Two:

A friend of mine had recently purchased a set of flower essences from Living Essences of Australia. She was showing the set to me and a few other friends. One friend, who had some major family issues surrounding forgiveness, decided to try the Black Kangaroo Paw, a flower essence. Black Kangaroo Paw is indicated for forgiveness and love. About five minutes after taking the remedy she started to cry uncontrollably for no apparent reason. This continued for at least ten minutes. She could not be consoled or calmed. I finally pulled out my bottle of Five Flower Formula (the Healing Herbs of England/FES version of Rescue Remedy), which I always carry with me, and gave her four drops—this calmed her almost immediately. The family issues dissipated after this. My friend was able to find the forgiveness she was seeking.

Case Number Three:

My wife and I took in a dog which had been abused. When we got her, she moped and was fairly listless. I prepared a combination of essences including Red Hibiscus for the emotional effects of past abuse; Comfrey to heal life's scars; Pink Tecoma for a sense of comfort, safety, and love; and Pale Pink Rose for transitions (all from Green Hope Farm). Over the next few days and weeks the dog completely changed into a playful, bold, and energetic dog. Although she is over four years old, people regularly assume she is a puppy.

Case Number Four:

An acupuncturist friend of mine asked for a recommendation for a patient of hers who was abused as a child and now walked around with a chip on his shoulder. He was always angry and bitter. He was tense and nasty. I suggested Mountain Devil from the Australian Bush line. My friend reported that she asked him to take it, not telling him what it was for. She left the room to get something, when she came back, he was smiling and appeared relaxed. She said the sweetness she knew was in him came out.

How to Use Flower Essences

One Flower Essence at a Time or a Combination of Flower Essences?

Flower essences can be used either way. A person can focus on one particular issue by using a single flower remedy or put together a mixture of flower essences to address a number of issues at once or different aspects of one issue.

Some flower essence lines, such as the Master's line, suggest the use of one flower essence at a time. Others say it is okay to combine anywhere from two to six well chosen essences. The most famous flower remedy of all, Bach's Rescue Remedy, is a combination of five different essences for any emergency, stressful, or traumatic situation. I think the best way to determine what works best for you is to experiment. I use flower essences both ways, singly and in combinations.

Are Flower Essences Just for Acute Situations?

Flower remedies can be used for acute situations, chronic states, and even "constitutionally." "Constitutionally" means to use a flower essence to address your overall mental/emotional state or to address a core issue in the person's being. Rather than addressing a particular issue, one identifies the single essence that seems to fit his or her personality, both the positive and negative attributes. The purpose here is for general balance.

Edward Bach identified twelve of his thirty-eight remedies as "personality type" remedies. He theorized that composite humanity is all twelve of these personality types. Individuals usually comprise one to three.

In her book *The Essential Flower Essence Handbook*, Lila Devi discusses the constitutional use of the Master's Flower Essences. She identifies the "theme" traits of these twenty essences.

In the book, *The Twelve Healers of the Zodiac* by Peter Damian, there is even the identification of the Bach Remedies based on astrological birth sign.

How to Take Flower Essences

Flower essences can be taken internally by directly dropping them in your mouth or by adding them to water or some other beverage. They can also be applied topically (directly, in oil, cream, or lotion). Flower essences are sturdy and tend not to be antidoted or neutralized by other substances.

To take flower essences, one can take three or four drops directly from the stock bottle or prepare a dosing bottle. A dosing bottle is made by filling a dropper bottle with spring water up to the shoulder of the bottle. You then add two droppers full of preserving agent (brandy, vodka, grain alcohol, glycerin, red shiso/vinegar). Next, put four drops of each flower essence in the bottle. Seal the bottle and succuss it (shake it while hitting it on the palm of your hand) at least ten times. Four drops is a dose. I recommend that for the first three days one takes a dose every two hours. After that, at least four times a day.

If you are applying the flower essences topically in oil, cream, or lotion, place four drops of each essence (from the original stock bottle) into the medium. Then succuss or stir the mixture.

Flower Essences and Other Forms of Healing

Flower Essences tend not to interfere with other types of remedies. They can generally be taken while one is on homeopathic remedies, herbs, or conventional medication. One exception would be if the preserving agent, such as alcohol, was contraindicated. If you have any concerns, you should discuss this with your health professional.

How to Use this Repertory

This repertory is designed to be a guide. It should help you to narrow the list of likely flower essences. To use it:

- Identify the issue or issues that you would like to address.
- Find the corresponding symptom(s) in the book.
- Read the annotations and jot down your short list of possible remedies, say three to ten.
- If you are not familiar with the remedies, go to the sources of the more detailed descriptions of the flower essences (refer to the bibliography in the back of the book for a list of these sources).
- Then select your remedy or remedies.

The codes that identify the makers of the flower remedies are as follows:

- Bach/English essences will be identified by a ● and are available through both the Bach company and FES (Healing Herbs).
- Master's Flower Essences will be identified by a ■.
- North American flower essences made by FES will be identified by a ▲.
- Green Hope Farm essences will be identified by a ▼.
- Australian Bush Essences will be identified by a ◆.
- Australian Living Essences will be identified by a ◗.
- Alaskan Flower Essences will be identified by a ❖.
- Pegasus essences will be identified by a ✚.
- Perelandra essences will be identified by a ✪.

MENTAL/EMOTIONAL
SYMPTOMS

Abandonment

Angelica ▲▼✚ — abandoned by spiritual world

Baby Blue Eyes ▲▼ — abandoned or rejected by father

Bleeding Heart ▲✚ — feeling abandoned in relationships

Chicory ●✚ — with neediness or manipulative behavior

Evening Primrose ▲ — rejected by mother in utero or early infancy

Grape ■ — feeling abandoned from loss

Holly ●✚ — masked with hostility, feelings of alienation

Mallow ▲▼✚ — difficulty making social contact

Maltese Cross ▼ — after violent, wrenching experiences

Mariposa Lilly ▲ — from lack of bonding with mother

Oregon Grape ▲ — expecting rejection, paranoia

Pink Monkeyflower ▲ — fearing abandonment with feelings of shame

Strawberry ■▲✚ — history of emotionally abusive parents

Sweet Chestnut ●✚ — feeling abandoned by God

Sweet Pea ▲ — social alienation and isolation

White Hibiscus ▼ — causing unconstructive behavior

Absent-Minded (see Concentration)

Abundance

Bog Blueberry ✽ — unconditional acceptance of abundance

Blueberry Pollen ✽ — releasing mental limitations to the experience of abundance

Buttercup ▲✚ — experiencing joy and abundance in the present

Crown of Thorns ✚ — "abundance is our birthright"

Forsythia ▲ — gateway to abundance

Harebell ✽ — manifesting abundance

Mesquite ✚ — opening oneself to pleasure and abundance

Money Plant ✚ — abundance, prosperity, earning money from what you love

Star Thistle-Yellow ✚ — for an inner sense of abundance

Abuse/Exploitation

Balsam Poplar ✽ — healing the impact of sexual abuse

Black Cohosh ▲ — in abusive, addictive relationships

● BACH — ■ MASTER'S — ▲ FES — ▼ GREEN HOPE — ◆ AUSTRALIAN BUSH
❿ LIVING/AUSTRALIA — ✽ ALASKAN — ✚ PEGASUS — ✪ PERELANDRA

Black-Eyed Susan ▲▼◆ — does not acknowledge prior abuse, repeats same pattern

Boab ◆ — release of abusive thought patterns from family

California Wild Rose ▲✛ — opens the heart to love and trust again after abuse

Centaury ● — those who accept abuse or exploitation

Cotton Grass ✤ — healing the effects of physical/sexual abuse

Dogwood ▲ — beaten, violated during childhood

Echinacea ▲✛ — extreme abuse and exploitation, need to restore dignity

Evening Primrose ▲ — abuse in utero or infancy

Golden Ear Drops ▲ — contact with prior abuse which was numbed or blotted out

Hibiscus ▲ — inability to feel sexual warmth or vitality

Impatiens ●✛ — anger and intolerance, may lead to violence or abuse

Mariposa Lily ▲ — abuse and abandonment from mother

Northern Lady's Slipper ✤ — healing the effects of physical abuse

Orange ■ — depression/despair/self-pity from past or present abuse

Pansy ▲✛ — to help acknowledge the effects of sexual abuse in one's life

Pine ● — emotional self-abuse/neglect from guilt, shaming or abuse

Pink Monkeyflower ▲ — abuse as a child or from sex partner, shame and guilt

Pink Yarrow ▲ — absorbing others' emotional violence, psychic toxicity/congestion

Pretty Face ▲ — beaten, violated, shamed, made to feel ugly or unwanted

Purple Monkeyflower ▲ — occult or ritual abuse

Red Hibiscus ▼ — connection to sexual self, healing from sexual abuse

River Beauty ✤ — recovery from emotional/sexual abuse

Rosemary ▲▼✛ — physical abuse leading to disconnection with physical body

Snapdragon ▲▼✛ — verbally abusive, biting, derogatory

Star of Bethlehem ●▼❯ — to soothe trauma of abuse

Strawberry ■▲✛ — history of emotionally abusive childhood

Sweet Chestnut ●✛ — severe abuse leading to deep despair and anguish

Tundra Twayblade ✤ — completely releasing impact of abuse

Vine ●✛ — compulsion to control/exploit other

● BACH — ■ MASTER'S — ▲ FES — ▼ GREEN HOPE — ◆ AUSTRALIAN BUSH
❯ LIVING/AUSTRALIA — ✤ ALASKAN — ✛ PEGASUS — ✪ PERELANDRA

White Yarrow ▼ — protection from psychic abuse

White Fireweed ❖ — recovery from emotional abuse

Wisteria ◆ — uncomfortable with sexuality from sexual abuse

Acceptance

Agrimony ●✚ — accepting painful feelings which are marked by cheerfulness

Almond ■▲✚ — accepting aging process

Alpine Lily ▲ — acceptance of the female body, especially reproductive organs

Apple ■▲✚ — healthy attitude, nourishing thoughts

Baby Blue Eyes ▲▼ — seeing innate goodness in others, especially when a cynic or bitter

Bauhinia ◆ — acceptance and open mindedness, embracing new concepts/ideas

Beech ●✚ — accepting differences when there is a tendency to be critical/judging

Bells of Ireland ▼✚ — accept and understand differences, combats prejudice

Billy Goat Plum ◆ — acceptance of one's physical body

Blackberry ■▲▼✚ — acceptance of change

Bleeding Heart ▲✚ — accepting others' need to be free in relationships

Brachycome ◗ — accepting others when one is critical

Buttercup ▲✚ — accepting own self-worth

Calendula ▲▼✚ — perceiving inner meaning of what others say, true listening

Cantaloupe ✚ — acceptance of higher self

Calla Lily ▲✚ — accepting sexual identity, when confused/ambivalent

Chrysanthemum ▲✚ — accepting mortality

Columbine ❖ — acceptance of one's unique and personal beauty

Correa ◗ — acceptance and learning from mistakes

Crab Apple ●▼✚ — accepting imperfection

Date ■ — receptivity, open mindedness

Endive ✚ — accepting health

Fairy Lantern ▲ — accepting responsibility of adulthood

Fawn Lily ▲ — acceptance of the mundane world, especially for those who retreat

---

● BACH — ■ MASTER'S — ▲ FES — ▼ GREEN HOPE — ◆ AUSTRALIAN BUSH
◗ LIVING/AUSTRALIA — ❖ ALASKAN — ✚ PEGASUS — ✪ PERELANDRA

Five Corners ◆ — love and acceptance of self, celebration of own beauty

Forget-Me-Not ▲◆✣ — accepting death of a loved one

Fuchsia ▲ — acceptance of repressed emotions

Golden Waitsia ◗ — accepting one's illness

Green Fairy Orchid ✣ — acceptance of the oneness of all creation

Hibbertia ◆ — acceptance of self and own innate knowledge

Holly ●✚ — compassion and understanding when one is jealous/hostile

Horseradish ✚ — accept bitterness in life and have courage to move on

Impatiens ●✚ — allowing others to have their own pace, letting life unfold

Jacob's Ladder ✣✚ — acceptance of the impulses of spirit

Love-Lies-Bleeding ▲ — acceptance of profound pain and suffering

Mallow ▲▼✚ — accepting aging process

Mustard ●✚ — accepting dark, painful emotions, working through depression

Oak ●✚ — accepting one's limits

Old Maid ✚ — acceptance/forgiveness of one's parents

Penstemon ▲✚ — inner strength to accept difficult circumstances

Philotheca ◆ — ability to accept praise, acknowledgement and love

Pincushion Hakea ◗ — accepting the beliefs of others

Pine ● — self-acceptance, releasing guilt and self-blame

Pink Monkeyflower ▲ — fear others will not accept one's deepest feelings

Pomegranate ▲▼✚ — acceptance of femininity

Ruta (Rue) ▲✚ — acceptance of oneself and one's true desires

Sage ▲✚ — understanding, learning from and accepting life experience

Saguaro ▲✚ — accepting legitimate authority and/or the wisdom of elders

Scotch Broom ▲✚ — accepting obstacles as opportunities

Sphagnum Moss ✣ — turning judgement into acceptance

Spiderwort ✚ — allows one to accept limitations

Spiraea ✣ — acceptance of support

Spruce ▲✚ — accepting one's own fallibility, willingness to compromise

Sunshine Wattle ◆ — acceptance of the beauty and joy in the present, optimism

Tiger Lily ▲✚ — self-appreciation and self-acceptance

● BACH — ■ MASTER'S — ▲ FES — ▼ GREEN HOPE — ◆ AUSTRALIAN BUSH
◗ LIVING/AUSTRALIA — ✣ ALASKAN — ✚ PEGASUS — ✪ PERELANDRA

Washington Lily ✚ — acceptance of spirituality

Yerba Buena ✚ — acceptance of the nature of God

Zinnia ▲▼✚✪ — accepting joy, willingness to laugh

Accident Prone

Jacaranda ◆ — lack of focused attention

Kangaroo Paw ◆ — awkward, clumsy

Pear ■▲▼✚ — returns a sense of rhythm and proportion

Red Lily ◆ — daydreaming

Impatiens ●✚ — impatient

Action

Aloe Vera ▲▼✚ — letting heart guide activity, especially when leads to burnout

Blackberry ■▲▼✚ — putting ideas into action, overcoming inertia

Cayenne ▲✚ — bring fiery impetus to slow-moving situations

Golden Yarrow ▲ — active/outgoing, despite sensitivity to environment/others

Hornbeam ● — overcoming resistance to daily responsibilities

Indian Pink ▲✚ — lifestyle with too much activity, ability to center self

Iris ▲ — stagnant creative forces

Mountain Pride ▲✚ — courageous action, taking a stand for one's beliefs

Sunflower ▲▼✚✿ — damaged male image/father relationship causing blockages

Tansy ▲✚ — taking decisive action, cutting through lethargy

Addiction

Agrimony ●✚ — drug abuse to appear cheerful, hiding true feelings

Almond ■▲✚ — over-indulgence in food or other substances

Angelica ▲▼✚ — useful during drug withdrawal

Arnica ▲✚ — repairing shock and trauma from drug abuse

Aspen ● — drug use to cover fear of the unknown, to dampen sensitivity

Baby Blue Eyes ▲▼ — drug use because the world is too harsh, no longer trusting

Basil ▲✚✪ — obsessive sexual promiscuity, sex and/or pornography addictions

---

● BACH — ■ MASTER'S — ▲ FES — ▼ GREEN HOPE — ◆ AUSTRALIAN BUSH
◗ LIVING/AUSTRALIA — ✿ ALASKAN — ✚ PEGASUS — ✪ PERELANDRA

Black Cohosh ▲ — in abusive/addictive relationships, co-dependent

Blue China Orchid ❱ — to strengthen will and take back control of self

California Poppy ▲▼ — tendency toward escapism, hallucinogenic drugs

Canyon Dudleya ▲ — compulsive seeking of spiritual or psychic highs

Chamomile ▲✚ — calming and stabilizing during drug withdrawal

Chaparral ▲✚ — cleansing of psychic toxins from drug abuse

Chestnut Bud ●✚ — breaking patterns/habits of addictive behavior

Chrysanthemum ▲✚ — drug/alcohol use from loss, deep fear of death/dying

Clematis ●✚ — drug use to escape from body/present time, especially psychedelic drugs

Dandelion ▲▼✚✤ — addiction to emotional pain

Endive ✚ — accepting health

Fairy Lantern ▲ — addiction as a form of escapism from responsibilities/adulthood

Golden Yarrow ▲ — drug use as a social barrier to dull sensitivity

Green Rein Orchid ✚ — to break co-dependent behavior

Lavender ▲✚ — sedating nerves from drug use, especially stimulants

Milkweed ▲✚ — use of opiates/sedative, inability to cope with ego/self

Morning Glory ▲▼✚ — breaking free of addictive habits, especially Stimulants

Mountain Pennyroyal ▲ — drug/alcohol abuse with psychic aberrations

Nicotiana ▲ — addiction to tobacco or any drug that numbs sensitivity

Olive ●✚ — depletion of mind/body from long term use of drugs/stimulants

Pale Corydalis ✤ — balances addictive and conditional patterns of loving

Peppermint ▲✚ — promoting a more awake state without stimulants

Pink Monkeyflower ▲ — drug use due to intolerable pain/sensitivity/shame

Plantain ▲ — children of alcoholics and drug addicts with immaturity/apprehension

Rescue Remedy (Five Flower Formula) ● — initial treatment, overdoses

Rosa Damascena Bifera (Damask Rose) ✚ — for addictive personality

Rosemary ▲▼✚ — drug use to sever connection with physical body

Sagebrush ▲✚ — letting go of old habits, emptiness/anxiety during withdrawal

● BACH — ■ MASTER'S — ▲ FES — ▼ GREEN HOPE — ◆ AUSTRALIAN BUSH
❱ LIVING/AUSTRALIA — ✤ ALASKAN — ✚ PEGASUS — ✪ PERELANDRA

Scarlet Monkeyflower ▲ — drug use to mask anger, powerlessness

Self-Heal ▲ — overall support in addiction therapy, for confidence in one's ability

Silver Princess Gum, Gungurra ❱ — perserverence to end an addiction

Star of Bethlehem ●▼❱ — burnout from drug abuse

Star Tulip ▲✚ — connection to spiritual self, especially drug use for false psychic states

Sunflower ▲▼✚✤ — low self-esteem associated with drug use

Tomato ■▼✚✪ — mental strength and courage during withdrawal

Adolescence

Alpine Lily ▲ — acceptance of one's female body during puberty

Angelica ▲▼✚ — protection of the soul during searching or experimentation

Baby Blue Eyes ▲▼ — cynicism, loss of innocence, disturbances with male figure

Basil ▲✚✪ — attraction to pornography/sexual conquest, integration of sexual self

Bleeding Heart ▲✚ — for crushes, broken heart

California Poppy ▲▼ — fascination with drugs/escapism

California Wild Rose ▲✚ — cynicism, apathy, alienation, suicidal feelings

Calla Lily ▲✚ — delayed puberty, confused sexual identity

Chamomile ▲✚ — rapid mood swings, emotional instability

Crab Apple ●▼✚ — self-disgust about acne, feeling ugly or impure

Fairy Lantern ▲ — delayed puberty, irregular/delayed menses (girls), overly feminine or delayed maturity (boys), anorexic tendencies

Gentian ●✚ — discouragement after academic/athletic/social setback

Golden Yarrow ▲ — shy and sensitive adolescents

Goldenrod ▲▼✚ — easily influenced by group pressure

Heather ●✚ — preoccupation with self, tendency to withdraw, masturbation

Holly ●✚ — feelings of jealousy, envy, rivalry

Larch ●✚ — confidence, voice changes in boys, integration of creative/sexual forces

Mallow ▲▼✚ — social insecurity, group pressures, trouble making/keeping friends

Manzanita ▲✚ — body issues, obsessive dieting, anorexia or bulimia

Mariposa Lily ▲ — stormy periods with mother/female figure, puberty too early

Mustard ●✚ — deep despair

Penstemon ▲✚ — feelings of not being "good enough"

Pink Monkeyflower ▲ — fear of expressing true feelings, fear of vulnerability

Pomegranate ▲▼✚ — creative development in girls, healthy attitude about menses

Pretty Face ▲ — feeling ugly or rejected, wanting beauty for social acceptance

Sagebrush ▲✚ — breaking old habits, maturity, individuation

Saguaro ▲✚ — extreme rebelliousness, resistance to authority figures

Sticky Monkeyflower ▲ — fear of intimacy leading to aggression or inhibition

Sunflower ▲▼✚❖ — conflict with father, masculine self, individuality

Sweet Pea ▲✚ — social alienation, family conflicts, gang behavior

Walnut ●✚ — courage to follow one's own convictions despite peer pressure

Wild Oat ● — confusion about life goals, direction, purpose

Willow ●✚ — resentment/bitterness, life not fair, blaming

Affection

Mountain Laurel ✚ — not loving yourself enough to receive affection

Aggression

Aggression Orchid ✚ — aggressive, impulsive, sexual aggression

Impatiens ●✚ — impatient and bossy

Larkspur ▲✚ — self-aggrandizement

Mountain Devil ◆ — hatred, jealousy, holding grudges, suspicion

Mountain Pride ▲✚ — strength and assertiveness in the face of adversary forces

Nicotiana ▲ — "macho," numbing feelings to appear strong

Oregon Grape ▲ — hostile, expecting aggression from others

Poison Oak ▲ — tendency to "fight" rather than "flight"

Snapdragon ▲▼✚ — verbal aggression and abuse

Sunflower ▲▼✚❖ — excessive egotism

Tiger Lily ▲✚ — overassertiveness, forced masculinity, feminine balance

---

● BACH — ■ MASTER'S — ▲ FES — ▼ GREEN HOPE — ◆ AUSTRALIAN BUSH
◗ LIVING/AUSTRALIA — ❖ ALASKAN — ✚ PEGASUS — ✪ PERELANDRA

Trillium ▲▼✦ — greed, lust for power

Trumpet Vine ▲✦ — lack of assertiveness, especially in speaking

Vine ●✦ — compulsion to be in control

Aging

Angel's Trumpet ▲✦ — spiritual surrender in dying process

Angelica ▲▼✦ — protection at threshold of death, during surgery, illness

Baby Blue Eyes ▲▼ — bitterness/cynicism, bringing childlike trust

Beech ●✦ — overly critical, inability to "forgive and forget"

Bleeding Heart ▲✦ — losing a mate/friend, going on in life

Buttercup ▲✦ — diminished self-esteem, feeling unworthy, valueless

California Wild Rose ▲✦ — for those prematurely occupied with the "other side"

Century Plant ▼ — dispelling notion that aging is natural or necessary

Centaury ● — sense of dignity and strength

Chicory ●✦ — needy, demanding, childish behavior

Chrysanthemum ▲✦ — confronting mortality, mid-life crisis

Clematis ●✦ — dreaminess, awareness moving in and out of body

Forget-Me-Not ▲✦❖ — transition during the dying process

Gentian ●✦ — pessimism/despair in the face of physical/health setbacks

Heather ●✦ — over-concern, pre-occupied with problems/worries

Hibiscus ▲ — to maintain sexual warmth/responsiveness during aging process

Holly ●✦ — opening heart, letting go of hostility, making peace

Honeysuckle ●✦ — dwells on the past, excessive nostalgia

Lavender ▲✦ — calming and soothing when agitated, difficulty sleeping

Madia ▲✦ — inability to concentrate or focus on details

Mallow ▲▼✦ — for the "crisis" of menopause

Mimulus ●✦ — numerous fears of everyday life, for shut-ins who do not take risks

Penstemon ▲✦ — courage to face obstacles, impediments, physical handicaps

Peppermint ▲✦ — for mental alertness, energizing thinking faculties

Pokeweed ✦ — for confidence and fear of aging, especially menopause

Pretty Face ▲ — over-identification with youthful appearance

Pumpkin ▼✚ — fear of aging

Purple Monkeyflower ▲ — uneasy/afraid due to out-of-body/spiritual experiences

Queen Anne's Lace ▲▼✚ — eliminates illusion of powerlessness

Rosemary ▲▼✚ — forgetful, drowsy

Sage ▲✚ — inner wisdom, insight/peace about meaning of life, serenity

St. John's Wort ▲▼✚ — lost connection to bodily functions, disturbed sleep

Self-Heal ▲ — confidence in own healing ability, over dependence on others

Star Tulip ▲✚ — shifting from physical to spiritual awareness

White Chestnut ● — chattering mind, breaking hold of obsessive thinking/worrying

Willow ●✚ — bitterness, blaming

Alienation

Alpine Lily ▲ — estranged from female body, deeper feminine self

Baby Blue Eyes ▲▼ — feeling that world is harsh, no longer trusting

Buttercup ▲✚ — not feeling worthy to others, or by worldly standards

California Wild Rose ▲✚ — apathy and indifference, suicidal tendencies

Calla Lily ▲✚ — alienation from sexual identity

Chrysanthemum ▲✚ — unable to accept death/dying

Evening Primrose ▲ — emotional distance, feeling rejected/unwanted

Fairy Lantern ▲ — fear of facing adulthood

Fawn Lily ▲ — reclusive soul, needy for perfection and an insulated environment

Golden Ear Drops ▲ — contacting painful childhood feelings

Grape ■ — "sour grapes" attitude

Lady's Slipper ▲ — self doubt with nervous depletion/sexual exhaustion

Manzanita ▲✚ — aversion to physical world and body

Mariposa Lily ▲ — estrangement from mother or the feminine, unloved/unwanted

Milkweed ▲✚ — separation/estrangement from core self

Poison Oak ▲ — discomfort with others, need for distance and space

Pretty Face ▲ — alienated from physical self

Saguaro ▲✚ — hostility toward authority figures, rebelliousness

Shooting Star ▲✚❖ — profound alienation

● BACH — ■ MASTER'S — ▲ FES — ▼ GREEN HOPE — ◆ AUSTRALIAN BUSH
◗ LIVING/AUSTRALIA — ❖ ALASKAN — ✚ PEGASUS — ✪ PERELANDRA

Spider Lily ▼✚ — for men who feel alienation towards women

Sunflower ▲▼✚✤ — disturbed relationship with father or father archetype in others

Sweet Pea ▲✚ — unconnected with family, community, land, fear of commitment

Tall Yellow Top ◆ — feeling lonely, isolated

Violet ▲ — feeling as if an outsider/stranger

Water Violet ●✚ — distancing oneself from others, seeing others as unworthy

Alignment

Paper Birch ✤ — alignment with one's true purpose

Ladies' Tresses ✤ — deep realignment with one's higher purpose

Cattail Pollen ✤ — alignment with the power of one's personal truth

Aloofness/Arrogance/Haughtiness

Baby Blue Eyes ▲▼ — aloofness with cynicism

California Wild Rose ▲✚ — aloofness as a form of apathy

Fawn Lily ▲ — fear of contamination or stress

Grape ■ — "sour grapes" attitude

Gymea Lily ◆ — arrogant, attention seeking, craving status/glamour, dominating

Larkspur ▲✚ — self-aggrandizement

Mallow ▲▼✚ — self-created barriers to friendship, lack of social warmth

Nasturtium ▲▼✚✪ — disdainful of social relationships

Nicotiana ▲ — for the loner who is emotionally unavailable/distant

Pink Monkeyflower ▲ — holding back for fear of rejection

Sunflower ▲▼✚✤ — distorted sense of self

Tansy ▲✚ — aloof, nonchalant with a lack of vitality

Violet ▲ — to create openness to others, especially in groups

Water Violet ●✚ — feeling separate with disdain or pride

Altruism

California Wild Rose ▲✚ — motivated, care about others and the earth

Chicory ●✚ — to promote selfless giving

● BACH — ■ MASTER'S — ▲ FES — ▼ GREEN HOPE — ◆ AUSTRALIAN BUSH
❱ LIVING/AUSTRALIA — ✤ ALASKAN — ✚ PEGASUS — ✪ PERELANDRA

Elm ●✚ — to balance heroic tendencies, overwhelmed, frustrated by responsibility

Heather ●✚ — stimulates compassion and altruism

Larkspur ▲✚ — joyful leadership for the good of all

Peach ■▲✚ — concern for the welfare of others, empathy

Tiger Lily ▲✚ — overcoming aggressiveness in work with others

Trillium ▲▼✚ — overcoming selfishness/greed

Ambition

Aloe Vera ▲▼✚ — workaholic tendencies, feeling burned out, depleted

Elm ●✚ — taking on too many responsibilities with overwhelm/over despondency

Larkspur ▲✚ — self-aggrandizement in leadership roles

Oak ●✚ — strong will, high goals pressing limits of endurance

Tiger Lily ▲✚ — overly masculine striving, competitive

Trillium ▲▼✚ — over concern with power and possessions

Vine ●✚ — obsession with power over others

Ambivalence

Alpine Lily ▲ — for women with difficulty accepting female body

California Wild Rose ▲✚ — lack of commitment, indifference to life

Calla Lily ▲✚ — confusion about sexual identity/expression of sexuality

Devil's Club ✤ — ambivalent about being on earth

Easter Lily ▲✚ — uncertainty about sexuality, feeling it may be impure

Evening Primrose ▲ — ambivalence about parenting/commitment from rejection

Fairy Lantern ▲ — inner conflict about growing up

Fawn Lily ▲ — conflict between inner peacefulness versus worldly involvement

Golden Yarrow ▲ — desire for social/artistic experiences, but too sensitive

Manzanita ▲✚ — aversion to physical body and world

Pomegranate ▲▼✚ — confused about choice of career and/or family life

Saguaro ▲✚ — conflict regarding authority figures, rebellion

Scleranthus ●✚ — difficulty in decision making, wavering between choices

Self-Heal ▲ — uncertainty about one's power to get well

● BACH — ■ MASTER'S — ▲ FES — ▼ GREEN HOPE — ◆ AUSTRALIAN BUSH
❱ LIVING/AUSTRALIA — ✤ ALASKAN — ✚ PEGASUS — ✪ PERELANDRA

Shooting Star ▲✚❖ — not fully accepting being on earth or part of humanity

Strawberry ■▲✚ — ungrounded, feeling unworthy

Violet ▲ — afraid of losing oneself in a group, shy, yet seeking social warmth

Anger

Barley ✚ — anger with sharp moodiness

Belladonna ✚ — constant anger

Black-Eyed Susan ▲▼◆ — repressed anger

Black Kangaroo Paw ◗ — grief/anger obsessive cycles

Blue Elf Viola ❖ — understanding/releasing anger through the heart

California Pitcher Plant ▲✚ — anger with denial

Century Agave ✚ — anger, impatience, sulking from immaturity

Chamomile ▲✚ — restoring calm when upset

Fireweed ▲❖✚ — transmute karma, remove anger, for Vietnam Vets

Feverfew ▲▼ — breaking up deep seated anger

Fuchsia ▲ — deep-seated anger that needs to be expressed

Fuchsia Grevillea ◗ — anger with underlying negativity, hypocrisy

Garlic ▲✚ — anger from hidden fear

Holly ●✚ — anger when love is thwarted or denied

Impatiens ●✚ — quick to anger

Jerusalem Artichoke ✚ — stimulates intellect, stabilizes mood

Kidney Bean ✚ — removes hidden anger

Mountain Devil ◆ — hatred, jealousy, holding grudges, suspicion

Orange Spiked Pea ◗ — for full expression, response, articulation without anger

Poison Oak ▲ — easily irritated, angry hostile

Rattlesnake Plantain Orchid ✚ — male aggression and anger

Red Leschenaultia ◗ — for couples/families with harshness/brittle attitudes

Scarlet Monkeyflower ▲ — fear of anger

Snapdragon ▲▼✚ — verbal aggression and abuse

Watermelon ▲✚ — "so angry unable to speak"

Willow ●✚ — bitterness, blaming, resentful

Ylang Ylang ✚ — calms anger, frustration, stress

● BACH — ■ MASTER'S — ▲ FES — ▼ GREEN HOPE — ◆ AUSTRALIAN BUSH
◗ LIVING/AUSTRALIA — ❖ ALASKAN — ✚ PEGASUS — ✪ PERELANDRA

Yucca ✚ — transforms anger/frustration into spiritual energy

Zucchini ▲▼✚❂ — release of frustration and anger

Anguish

Love-Lies-Bleeding ▲ — profound anguish

Sweet Chestnut ●✚ — experiencing the "dark night of the soul"

Animal and Animal Care

Animal Emergency Care ▼ — rescue remedy for animals

Arnica ▲✚ — shock, trauma, illness, injury, surgery

Aspen ● — unknown fear/terror, especially for wild or nervous animals

Bleeding Heart ▲✚ — pets who whine or mope until owner returns

Borage ▲▼✚ — depression from illness or old age

Chamomile ▲✚ — barking dogs, emotional upset with stomach distress

Cherry Plum ●✚ — extreme tension/stress, such as a trapped animal

Chestnut Bud ●✚ — to instill effective learning patterns during training

Chicory ●✚ — whining puppies or kittens, feigning illness for attention

Cosmos ▲▼✚ — inter-species communication

Dill ▲▼❂ — overwhelm/confusion, eg. travel or schedule upset

Flee Free ▼ — for fleas and other pests

Forget-Me-Not ▲✚✤ — transition during the dying process

Grape ■ — neglected, abandoned pets, animals on own too much, loners, loss of companion/owner

Holly ●✚ — jealous pets, especially jealous of another pet

Impatiens ●✚ — nervous, high strung, impulsive animals

Larkspur ▲✚ — allows a closer affinity for those working with animals

Love-Lies-Bleeding ▲ — wounded/suffering animals

Mariposa Lily ▲ — mother-infant bonding, especially surrogate, pet in a new home

Mimulus ●✚ — nervous, jittery, shy animals

Pear ■▲▼✚ — for any troubling experience or emergency: accidents, shock, etc.

Penstemon ▲✚ — illness or trauma, gives inner strength

Pink Yarrow ▲ — pets who mirror caretakers' emotions

Quaking Grass ▲✚ — group/herd animals living together

Red Clover ▲▼ — calming hysterical animals, especially cats

Rescue Remedy (Five Flower Formula) ● — any stress or emergency

---

● BACH — ■ MASTER'S — ▲ FES — ▼ GREEN HOPE — ◆ AUSTRALIAN BUSH
❱ LIVING/AUSTRALIA — ✤ ALASKAN — ✚ PEGASUS — ❂ PERELANDRA

Self-Heal ▲ — stimulates inner healing forces, awakens vitality and will to live

Snapdragon ▲▼✚ — for animals who bite, are aggressive

Spinach ■ — stress of domesticated/new household, poor weaning

Star of Bethlehem ●▼❱ — abused, injured, traumatized animals

Tiger Lily ▲✚ — for hostile or aggressive cats or dogs

Tomato ■▼✚✪ — fearful, skiddish animals

Vervain ●✚ — for hyperactive, overly tense animals

Vine ●✚ — animals which dominate younger/weaker animals

Walnut ●✚ — before and after a major move, also good for animals giving birth

Wild Rose ● — for apathetic, listless animals

Anxiety

Aspen ● — anxiety that has no reason

Balm-Lemon ✚ — calms and represses anxiety

Banana ■▲▼✚ — anxiety from clouded judgement, loss of perspective

Basil ▲✚✪ — eases anxiety by getting to the core of the cause

Bells of Ireland ▼✚ — eases stress and anxiety

Bottlebrush ▼◆✚ — general sense of anxiety, especially with body twitches/ticks

Cerato ●✚ — excessive anxiety about failure, depending on others for advice

Chamomile ▲✚ — calming overly anxious states

Chrysanthemum ▲✚ — morbid thoughts or suppression of thoughts of own death

Elm ●✚ — overstriving for perfection, fear that one will disappoint

Figwort ✚ — for agitated anxiety

Filaree ▲✚ — worry/concern about trivial problems of daily life

Forget-Me-Not ▲✚✤ — anxiety with paranoia

Garlic ▲✚ — chronic anxiety/worry, ghostly countenance

Ginseng ✚ — sexual anxiety

Golden Yarrow ▲ — performance anxiety, especially felt in solar plexus

Golden Waitsia ❱ — anxiety associated with perfectionism

Goldenrod ▲▼✚ — needing social approval, unsure of one's own value

Jacob's Ladder ✤✚ — anxiety with a history of incest with father

Khat ✚ — anxiety over aging

Larch ●✚ — fear of failure, paralyzed by anxiety

Mimulus ●✚ — anxiety/nervousness about daily life, fretful, timid

Mustard ●✚ — free floating anxiety, especially with depression

Nicotiana ▲ — coping with anxiety by anesthetizing emotions, a cool exterior

Pepper ✚ — general anxiety

Pink Monkeyflower ▲ — anxiety that others will not accept you, shame or guilt

Poison Ivy ▲✚ — anxiety with irritability

Pretty Face ▲ — anxiety about physical appearance

Prickly Pear Cactus ▲✚ — anxiety in a relationship

Purple Flag Flower ◗ — anxiety from pressure and tension

Pyrethrum ✚ — anxiety causing paranoia

Red Chestnut ●✚ — anxiety about others

Rose-Honorine De Brabant ✚ — for elimination of stress, hysteria, and anxiety

Sweet Flag ✚ — extreme anxiety, stress, fear

Tomato ■▼✚○ — anxiety from fear and weakness

Trumpet Vine ▲✚ — anxiety and fear which blocks expressiveness

Wooly Smokebush ◗ — anxiety associated with self-importance

Apathy

Blackberry ■▲▼✚ — connect with will

California Wild Rose ▲✚ — indifference to life

Gorse ●✚ — encourages hope in those who have given up

Kapok Bush ◆ — resignation, easily discouraged

Orange ■ — apathy with melancholy

Peppermint ▲✚ — apathetic thinking, mental sluggishness

Tansy ▲✚ — apparent laziness, stagnant energy, overly phlegmatic

Tulip ✚ — disinterested in day-to-day life

Wild Rose ● — lacking motivation to get well, especially with lingering illness

Aphrodisiac

Avocado ■▲▼✚ — brings forward feelings

Mullein ▲✚ — invigorates male virility

Papaya ▲▼✚ — unity of mind, clarity of conscience in a relationship

---

● BACH — ■ MASTER'S — ▲ FES — ▼ GREEN HOPE — ◆ AUSTRALIAN BUSH
◗ LIVING/AUSTRALIA — ✤ ALASKAN — ✚ PEGASUS — ○ PERELANDRA

Persimmon ▲✚ — extremely potent aphrodisiac, especially for women

Petunia ▲✚ — increases blood flow (applied topically)

Pomegranate ▲▼✚ — "love potion" for women

Ruta (Rue) ▲✚ — strengthens emotions and sensitivity

Spice Bush ▲✚ — increases sense of pleasure (applied topically)

Watermelon ▲✚ — stimulates fertility in female, potency in male

Appreciation

Brachycome ◗ — appreciation and respect for the intrinsic value of others

Bougainvillaea ▼✚ — appreciation of grace and beauty

Buttercup ▲✚ — recognizing self-worth, having gifts to share with others

Calendula ▲▼✚ — perceiving inner meaning of what others say

California Wild Rose ▲✚ — joy and appreciation of life

Dogwood ▲ — appreciation of beauty

Holly ●✚ — ability to feel joy and happiness for others

Manzanita ▲✚ — appreciation of the body as the "temple of the spirit"

Oregon Grape ▲ — seeing the good hearted intentions of others

Peach ■▲✚ — considerate, giving

Peony ▲✚ — appreciation of others

Quaking Grass ▲✚ — appreciation for the worth of others in group work

Sage ▲✚ — appreciating the lessons of life, learning/growing from life experiences

Sassafras ✚ — appreciation of the divine in all of us

Snakevine ◗ — brings back confidence/appreciation of achievements

Spinach ■ — childlike joy

Valerian ▲✚ — appreciation of life

Water Violet ●✚ — appreciation of social relationships

Argumentative

Banana ■▲▼✚ — quarrelsome, false pride, need for recognition

Bayberry ✚ — refusing to listen to another's point of view

Calendula ▲▼✚ — using sharp and cutting words

Dagger Hakea ◆ — resentment, bitterness toward family, friends, lovers

Eucalyptus ▲✚ — to understand the other's position

● BACH — ■ MASTER'S — ▲ FES — ▼ GREEN HOPE — ◆ AUSTRALIAN BUSH
◗ LIVING/AUSTRALIA — ❖ ALASKAN — ✚ PEGASUS — ✪ PERELANDRA

Hibiscus ▲ — for those who like to argue and fight all the time
Isopogon ◆ — stubborn and controlling
Lavender ▲✚ — calming and soothing when agitated
Purple and Red Kangaroo Paw ◗ — relationships with circular arguments of blame

Arrogance (see Aloofness)

Assertiveness

Banksia Marginata ✚ — assertiveness in issues of sexuality
Geraldton Wax ◗ — strength not to be pressured against one's will
Goddess Grasstree ◗ — not being emotionally dependent
Holly ●✚ — peace loving, yet assertive
Hybrid Pink Fairy/Cowslip Orchid ◗ — not caught up in praise/condemnation
Motherwort ✚ — setting of healthy boundaries
Mountain Pride ▲✚ — courage and strength when facing overwhelming challenges
Parakeelya ◗ — self-esteem and assertiveness
Trumpet Vine ▲✚ — assertiveness in speech

Attachment

Angel's Trumpet ▲✚ — soul too attached to body during dying process
Banana ■▲▼✚ — negative attachments
Bleeding Heart ▲✚ — holding on to others, emotional possessiveness
Bunchberry ✤ — moving beyond one's attachment to distraction
Canyon Dudleya ▲ — inflating/exaggerating ordinary events
Chicory ●✚ — obsessive need for attention in relationships
Chrysanthemum ▲✚ — over-identification with fame/fortune, earthly life
Cotton Grass ✤ — release of shock and trauma
Honeysuckle ●✚ — dwells on the past, excessive nostalgia
Love-Lies-Bleeding ▲ — over-personalization of one's pain/suffering
Morning Glory ▲▼✚ — holding on to destructive habits, addictions
Oak ●✚ — holding on to struggle, not knowing when to let go
Red Chestnut ●✚ — over-concern and obsessive worry for others
River Beauty ✤ — washing away the old, allowing the new to come in
Round-Leaved Sundew ✤ — releasing inappropriate ego attachment

● BACH — ■ MASTER'S — ▲ FES — ▼ GREEN HOPE — ◆ AUSTRALIAN BUSH
◗ LIVING/AUSTRALIA — ✤ ALASKAN — ✚ PEGASUS — ✪ PERELANDRA

Sage ▲✚ — appropriate detachment as part of aging process, larger soul perspective

Sagebrush ▲✚ — holding on to false identity/life circumstances

Sweetgale ❖ — releasing emotional blockages

Trillium ▲▼✚ — greedy attachment to possession and/or power

Attention

Avocado ■▲▼✚ — missing details, "out to lunch"

Chicory ●✚ — obsessive need for attention

Clematis ●✚ — being in the here-and-now

Goldenrod ▲▼✚ — seeking negative attention

Heather ●✚ — drawing attention to oneself by talking about one's problems

Madia ▲✚ — inability to concentrate or focus on details

Pink Monkeyflower ▲ — avoiding social attention, wanting to hide or cover up

Queen Anne's Lace ▲▼✚ — to focus and clarify psychic forces

Rabbitbrush ▲✚ — attention to details while maintaining overview of big picture

Authority

Black Kangaroo Paw ◗ — resentment of parents, other authority figures growing up

Centaury ● — over-dependence on authority of others, subservient "doormat"

Cerato ●✚ — for those who rely on the authority of others to decide what is true

Fairy Lantern ▲ — childlike dependence/helplessness

Iris ▲ — coming in to personal power, being your own authority

Lady's Slipper ▲ — estrangement from inner authority

Purple Monkeyflower ▲ — fear of spiritual authority

Red Helmet Orchid ◆ — rebellious, problems with authority

Sage ▲✚ — elder wisdom

Saguaro ▲✚ — conflict regarding authority figures, rebellion

Snapdragon ▲▼✚ — verbal bullying and abuse

Sunflower ▲▼✚❖ — conflict involving father or father figures

Vine ●✚ — overly imposing authority on others

● BACH — ■ MASTER'S — ▲ FES — ▼ GREEN HOPE — ◆ AUSTRALIAN BUSH
◗ LIVING/AUSTRALIA — ❖ ALASKAN — ✚ PEGASUS — ◯ PERELANDRA

Walnut ●✚ — independence from authority of others, charting one's own path

Watermelon ▲✚ — fear of authority

Avoidance

Agrimony ●✚ — wearing a cheerful mask to hide painful emotions

Black-Eyed Susan ▲▼◆ — not acknowledging dark emotions

Canyon Dudleya ▲ — wishing to escape daily events and ordinary reality

Christmas Tree (Kanya) ❱ — those who avoid family responsibilities/chores

Chrysanthemum ▲✚ — denial or avoidance of one's mortality

Clematis ●✚ — escape from the present by daydreaming of what the future is

Coconut ■ — making excuses, escapism, avoidance of "tests," a quitter

Evening Primrose ▲ — sexual/emotional repression from childhood abuse/rejection

Fairy Lantern ▲ — avoiding full adult identity and responsibilities

Fuchsia ▲ — repressing basic emotions, covering with superficial emotionality

Honeysuckle ●✚ — escapes present by dwelling on the past

Nicotiana ▲ — false persona of toughness/strength to avoid real feelings

Pink Monkeyflower ▲ — fear of deepest feelings, profound feelings of shame

Poison Oak ▲ — creating distance by erecting hostile or offensive barriers

Scarlet Monkeyflower ▲ — fear of anger or strong emotions

Water Violet ●✚ — refraining from social contact out of feeling superior

Awakeness

Chestnut Bud ●✚ — to observe one's experience clearly and learn from it

Clematis ●✚ — to be fully present/wakeful, especially with tendency is to float/drift away

Cosmos ▲▼✚ — integrating thoughts with speech, to speak and think with clarity

Dill ▲▼✪ — nervous overwhelm form too many sensations/experiences

Milkweed ▲✚ — inability to cope with awake states of consciousness

Morning Glory ▲▼✛ — awakening life energy without the need for stimulants

Peppermint ▲✛ — stimulates healthy mental alertness

Rabbitbrush ▲✛ — ability to handle many diverse activities with clear attention

Rosemary ▲▼✛ — forgetful, drowsy

St. John's Wort ▲▼✛ — those overly expanded into a dream-like consciousness

Awareness

Alder ✤ — awareness beyond our normal range of perception

Angelica ▲▼✛ — attunement to higher worlds for guidance/protection

Avocado ■▲▼✛ — greater awareness and mental focus

Black-Eyed Susan ▲▼◆ — penetrating insight into emotions

Bladderwort ✤ — awareness of illusion

Bougainvillaea ▼✛ — awareness of grace and beauty in life

Calendula ▲▼✛ — sensitivity to the meaning of what others say

Chaparral ▲✛ — psychic cleansing of disturbing images

Chestnut Bud ●✛ — learning from past experience, not repeating mistakes

Chives ▼✪ — awareness of internal masculine and feminine energies

Coconut ■ — super-consciousness

Comandra ✤ — awareness of connection to the plant kingdom

Cosmos ▲▼✛ — bringing higher thought into spoken word, mental awareness

Crowberry ✤ — awareness/acceptance of cycles of light and darkness

Dandelion ▲▼✛✤ — awareness of emotional tension in the body

Forget-Me-Not ▲✛✤ — recognizing connection to the spiritual world

Fuchsia ▲ — bringing repressed emotions to the surface

Ginseng ✛ — developing spiritual awareness

Golden Ear Drops ▲ — contacting painful childhood feelings

Hairy Butterwort ✤ — awareness of support/guidance from higher realms

Lady's Slipper ▲✤ — awareness of subtle energy flows for healing

Lavender ▲✛ — highly refined awareness

Love-Lies-Bleeding ▲ — awareness of one's suffering

Madia ▲✛ — mental clarity and concentration

● BACH — ■ MASTER'S — ▲ FES — ▼ GREEN HOPE — ◆ AUSTRALIAN BUSH
◗ LIVING/AUSTRALIA — ✤ ALASKAN — ✛ PEGASUS — ✪ PERELANDRA

Manzanita ▲✚ — awareness of the physical body and world

Maple ✚ — awareness of essential wholeness

Money Plant ✚ — awareness of the healing power of the mind

Monkshood ▲✚✤ — awareness of true self

Mugwort ▲✚ — awareness during dreaming, greater psychic sensitivity

Mullein ▲✚ — awareness of "inner voice"

Nootka Lupine ✤ — where awareness needs to be focused in order to make change

Northern Twayblade ✤ — awareness of spiritual consciousness

One-Sided Wintergreen ✤ — awareness of how one's energy affects others

Paper Birch ✤ — awareness of one's true purpose

Pineapple Weed ✤ — awareness of self and surroundings, harmony between mothers and children and between humans and the earth

Queen Anne's Lace ▲▼✚ — balanced psychic awareness, especially with distorted clarity

Rabbitbrush ▲✚ — seeing the big picture

Sage ▲✚ — inner wisdom of life experiences, understanding meaning of life

Sagebrush ▲✚ — deep awareness of inner self

Scarlet Monkeyflower ▲ — awareness of powerful emotions, anger

Shasta Daisy ▲ — synthesizing many diverse ideas into a unified whole

Shooting Star ▲✚✤ — astrological awareness

Single Delight ✤ — awareness of the omnipresence of light

Spiraea ✤ — awareness of support/nurturing from nature

Star Tulip ▲✚ — greater receptivity to subtle states of awareness

Tamarack ✤ — awareness of true essence, self-confidence/understanding abilities

Yarrow ▲ — compassionate awareness

Yellow Dryas ✤ — awareness of self and family during times of growth/expansion

Yerba Santa ▲✚ — recognition of repressed emotional pain

Awkwardness

Dogwood ▲ — emotional trauma stored in body, leading to awkwardness

Lobelia ✚ — feeling awkward and clumsy

Mallow ▲▼✚ — discomfort in social situations, fear of reaching out to others

Manzanita ▲✚ — alienation from physical body and world

Pink Monkeyflower ▲ — social insecurity due to shame, fear of exposure

Pretty Face ▲ — feeling awkward due to physical appearance

Shooting Star ▲✚❖ — feeling alien and out of place

Sticky Monkeyflower ▲ — unease with sexuality, leading to avoidance or aggression

Violet ▲ — afraid of losing oneself in a group, shy

Bad Luck

Four Leaf Clover ✚ — increases practical, logical thinking and intuition

Pink Impatiens ◗ — for those who feel unlucky in the ideals for which they strive

Balance

Almond ■▲✚ — to avoid "burning the candle at both ends"

Apple ■▲✚ — healthy attitude, nourishing thoughts

Balsam Poplar ❖ — balancing sexual energy in the body

California Poppy ▲▼ — balance in inner development

Calla Lily ▲✚ — balancing one's male and female aspects

Corn ■▲▼✚✪ — spirituality to both heaven/earth, physical body/psychic awareness

Fawn Lily ▲ — balance between inner spirituality and outer commitment

Goldenrod ▲▼✚ — balance between "group" consciousness and individual awareness

Green Fairy Orchid ❖ — balancing male and female energies in the heart

Hops Bush ◗ — balancing scattered energy

Labrador Tea ❖ — moving from an unbalanced state to a centered, energized state

Lamb's Quarters ❖ — balance between the heart and mind

Lotus ▲✚ — balanced spirituality

Morning Glory ▲▼✚ — balance and regularity in daily habits and lifestyle

---

● BACH — ■ MASTER'S — ▲ FES — ▼ GREEN HOPE — ◆ AUSTRALIAN BUSH
◗ LIVING/AUSTRALIA — ❖ ALASKAN — ✚ PEGASUS — ✪ PERELANDRA

Mugwort ▲✚ — to balance the psychic life, daytime/nighttime consciousness

Nasturtium ▲▼✚❂ — balance after over worry and intense mental activity

Nicotiana ▲ — to balance heart forces

Pear ■▲▼✚ — returns a sense of rhythm and proportion

Pomegranate ▲▼✚ — to balance female creativity, inner/outer, creative/procreative

Queen Anne's Lace ▲▼✚ — to harmonize emerging psychic faculties

Quince ▲✚ — balancing the soul's need to express both power and love

Scleranthus ●✚ — extreme instability and imbalance, restlessness and confusion

Shooting Star ▲✚✤ — balance between the celestial and the physical

Sitka Spruce Pollen ✤ — balancing power and gentleness

Soapberry ✤ — balancing one's personal power with the power of nature

Sunflower ▲▼✚✤ — balance between self-effacement and self-aggrandizement

Opium Poppy ✤ — balancing activity and rest, evolution and being

Twinflower ✤ — balancing listening and speaking skills

Vervain ●✚ — to bring inner equanimity and moderation

White Spruce ✤ — balance of logic and intuition

Barriers/Boundaries

Evening Primrose ▲ — lack of emotional presence from rejection in infancy

Fawn Lily ▲ — naturally reclusive, protecting oneself from too much social contact

Fig ■▲✚ — barriers from rigidity, tension, difficulty with change

Goldenrod ▲▼✚ — creating barriers through antisocial or obnoxious behavior

Mallow ▲▼✚ — creating barriers to friendships

Monkshood ▲✚✤ — lack of boundaries from a weak spiritual identity

One-Sided Wintergreen ✤ — boundaries in alignment with one's highest truth

Onion ▲✚ — releases toxic emotions and mental barriers

Penstemon ▲✚ — strength and courage to overcome obstacles

● BACH — ■ MASTER'S — ▲ FES — ▼ GREEN HOPE — ◆ AUSTRALIAN BUSH
◗ LIVING/AUSTRALIA — ✤ ALASKAN — ✚ PEGASUS — ❂ PERELANDRA

Pink Monkeyflower ▲ — barriers because of shame/unworthiness/vulnerability

Poison Oak ▲ — creating distance by erecting hostile or offensive barriers

Rock Water ● — barriers from rigidity, self-discipline or asceticism

Star Tulip ▲✚ — barrier in relationship to higher self

Walnut ●✚ — breaking through limits from past associations and influences

Water Violet ●✚ — feeling distant and aloof, especially from pride

White Violet ❖ — appropriate boundaries from divine trust

Bereavement (see Grief)

Blame

Baby Blue Eyes ▲▼ — blame tinged with cynicism

Beech ●✚ — blame with critical judgement of others

Correa ◗ — acceptance and learning from mistakes without blame or resentment

Grape ■ — "sour grapes" attitude

Green Rose ✚◗ — grief with stagnation, repetition of mistakes

Hyssop ▲▼✚ — releasing feelings of guilt and blame

Larch ●✚ — self-blame when making errors, leading to unwillingness to take risks

Oregon Grape ▲ — expecting blame or negativity from others

Pine ● — self-blame, hard on oneself, filled with guilt feelings

Pink Yarrow ▲ — absorbing others' feelings of blame, emotional projection

Purple and Red Kangaroo Paw ◗ — relationships with circular arguments of blame

Raspberry ■✚ — with touchy nature, taking things personally, overreacting

Sage ▲✚ — blaming others/circumstances for life destiny

Saguaro ▲✚ — blaming authority figures for personal and world problems

Snapdragon ▲▼✚ — verbal criticism and abuse

Willow ●✚ — bitterness, blaming, resentful

Zinnia ▲▼✚✪ — bitterness/resentment, blaming others, life is not fair, feel wronged

---

● BACH — ■ MASTER'S — ▲ FES — ▼ GREEN HOPE — ◆ AUSTRALIAN BUSH
◗ LIVING/AUSTRALIA — ❖ ALASKAN — ✚ PEGASUS — ✪ PERELANDRA

Bonding

Bottlebrush ▼◆✚ — bonding between mother and child

Gum Plant ▲✚ — bonding between individuals

Mariposa Lily ▲ — mother-infant bonding, especially surrogate, pet in a new home

Noni ▲ — to prepare women for childbearing and motherhood

Plumeria ✚ — bonding with family

Watermelon ▲✚ — bonding between couples wanting to get pregnant

Breakthrough

Black-Eyed Susan ▲▼◆ — breakthrough of self-awareness

Blackberry ■▲▼✚ — ability to put thoughts into action, manifestation

Cayenne ▲✚ — overcome inertia and move decisively to next step

Fuchsia ▲ — bringing repressed emotions to the surface

Indian Paintbrush ▲✚ — ability to rouse vital forces for creative work

Iris ▲ — to overcome creative blocks when lacking inspiration

Morning Glory ▲▼✚ — overcoming depleting habit patterns, catalyzing fresh forces

Mountain Pride ▲✚ — courage and strength when facing overwhelming challenges

Rescue Remedy (Five Flower Formula) ● — to call on inner resources during stress

Sagebrush ▲✚ — letting go of "old baggage," ability to take next step

Scarlet Monkeyflower ▲ — to bring repressed emotions/fear of anger to awareness

Scleranthus ●✚ — to come to a decision after wavering

Tansy ▲✚ — decisive action, overcoming lethargy and procrastination

Walnut ●✚ — breaking through limits from past associations and influences

Brokenheartedness

Angelica ▲▼✚ — transcending relationships as the only source of fulfillment

Bleeding Heart ▲✚ — emotional detachment/acceptance with end of a relationship

Borage ▲▼✚ — cheerful courage and upliftment, to ease pain, constriction, grief

Boronia ◆ — pining for recently ended relationships

California Wild Rose ▲✚ — acceptance of painful feelings in the heart

Chamomile ▲✚ — calming emotional trauma, argumentativeness in relationships

Forget-Me-Not ▲✚❖ — opens the heart to spiritual realms, especially after a death

Hawthorne ✚ — for broken romances

Helleborus-Black ✚ — depression after a broken romance

Holly ●✚ — opening heart to true love and acceptance, compassion

Honeysuckle ●✚ — escapes present by dwelling on the past

Love-Lies-Bleeding ▲ — to learn compassion from one's suffering

Pink Monkeyflower ▲ — to retain trust and vulnerability despite prior heartbreak

Strawberry ■▲✚ — for grounding, sense of self-worth after a break-up

Sweet Chestnut ●✚ — experiencing the "dark night of the soul"

Yerba Santa ▲✚ — deep-seated pain/trauma which blocks the heart

Burn-Out

Aloe Vera ▲▼✚ — workaholic tendencies, feeling burned out, depleted

Cowkicks ◗ — re-energizing

Gorse ●✚ — encourages hope in those who have burned-out

Kolokoltchik ◗ — rekindles the strength of endurance

Lavender ▲✚ — soothing frayed, overstimulated nerves

Leafless Orchid ◗ — feelings of depletion for those who work in service to others

Macrocarpa ◆ — renews enthusiasm

Orange ■ — feeling burdened

Papaya ▲▼✚ — clears mental confusion and tension

Pink Everlasting ◗ — burn-out of the heart

Purple Nightshade ✚ — soothes jangled, burned-out nervous states

Red Beak Orchid ◗ — renews energy and inspiration

Spinach ■ — feeling burdened, overwhelmed with mild distrust to paranoia

White Spider Orchid ◗ — brings love and caring to darkest corners of the world

Calm

Agrimony ●✚ — false outer calm, hiding inner conflict

● BACH — ■ MASTER'S — ▲ FES — ▼ GREEN HOPE — ◆ AUSTRALIAN BUSH
◗ LIVING/AUSTRALIA — ❖ ALASKAN — ✚ PEGASUS — ✪ PERELANDRA

Almond ■▲✚ — when "burning the candle at both ends"

Angel's Trumpet ▲✚ — deep peacefulness in the soul around dying process

Banana ■▲▼✚ — ability to step back and observe

Bluebell ◆ — feeling like you are going to fall apart

Canyon Dudleya ▲ — over excitement, dramatization, desire for intense experiences

Chamomile ▲✚ — fretful, fussy, tension — especially felt in stomach region

Cosmos ▲▼✚ — to harmonize an overly active mind when many ideas flood it

Daisy ✚ — calm when overwhelmed

Dog Rose of the Wild Forces ◆ — calm/centered during turmoil

Filaree ▲✚ — letting go of worries and anxieties that limit participation in life

Garlic ▲✚ — release of nervous fears and insecurities

Indian Pink ▲✚ — remaining calm and centered in the midst of intense activity

Larch ●✚ — fearful of making a mistake

Lavender ▲✚ — soothing frayed, overstimulated nerves

Lettuce ■✚ — for inner quietude, restlessness, too many thoughts

Licorice ✚ — calms restlessness, insomnia

Lotus ▲✚ — purifies emotions

Many Headed Dryandra ◗ — calms, strengthens, inspires for stability and fulfillment

Marjoram ✚ — calms, soothes, comforts and protects from harm

Mimulus ●✚ — calming anxiety/nervousness about daily life

Mint Bush ◆ — calmness and clarity, ability to cope

Nicotiana ▲ — false appearance of calm, using tobacco to calm

Petunia ▲✚ — feeling calm, sure, aware of what is most important

Pink Yarrow ▲ — tendency to be an emotional sponge

Purple Monkeyflower ▲ — fear of the occult, calm during spiritual experiences

Purple Nightshade ✚ — soothes jangled, burned-out nervous states

Red Chestnut ●✚ — releasing over-concern and obsessive worry for others

Red Clover ▲▼ — panic and group hysteria

● BACH — ■ MASTER'S — ▲ FES — ▼ GREEN HOPE — ◆ AUSTRALIAN BUSH
◗ LIVING/AUSTRALIA — ❖ ALASKAN — ✚ PEGASUS — ✪ PERELANDRA

Rescue Remedy (Five Flower Formula) ● — immediate calming in accidents

Star of Bethlehem ●▼▶ — soothe effects of shock or trauma

Valerian ▲✚ — promotes relaxation

White Chestnut ● — constant churning and over activity of the mind

Yellow Flag Flower ▶ — lightheartedness/calmness despite rising tension/pressure

Caring (see Compassion)

Catalyst

Black-Eyed Susan ▲▼◆ — insight into emotions where there has been lack

Blackberry ■▲▼✚ — ability to put thoughts into action, manifestation

Cayenne ▲✚ — overcome inertia and move decisively to next step

Fireweed ▲❖✚ — transformation catalyst which leads towards new phase

Fuchsia ▲ — catalyst which brings repressed emotions to the surface

Indian Paintbrush ▲✚ — ability to rouse vital forces for creative work

Peach ■▲✚ — a catalyst for all forms of healing

Self-Heal ▲ — stimulates inner healing forces, awakens vitality and will to live

Tansy ▲✚ — decisive action, overcoming lethargy and procrastination

Catharsis

Black Cohosh ▲ — ability to confront abusive or destructive forces

Black-Eyed Susan ▲▼◆ — release of hidden emotions through understanding/insight

Cayenne ▲✚ — promoting catharsis by bringing more fiery stimulus to stagnancy

Chaparral ▲✚ — psychic cleansing of disturbing images

Evening Primrose ▲ — healing trauma from in utero/infancy

Fuchsia ▲ — release of repressed emotions

Golden Ear Drops ▲ — release of painful childhood memories

Holly ●✚ — release of hostility/anger from unknown cause

Hooded Ladies Tresses ✚ — catharsis to attain a higher state

Love-Lies-Bleeding ▲ — transcendence and insight from one's suffering

---

● BACH — ■ MASTER'S — ▲ FES — ▼ GREEN HOPE — ◆ AUSTRALIAN BUSH
▶ LIVING/AUSTRALIA — ❖ ALASKAN — ✚ PEGASUS — ✪ PERELANDRA

Scarlet Monkeyflower ▲ — release of powerful emotions, especially anger

Willow ●✚ — release of anger, blame, resentment

Centeredness

Angelica ▲▼✚ — spiritual centeredness

Bistort ▲✚ — to remain centered and fully present

Broccoli ▲▼✪ — staying centered when under attack

Canyon Dudleya ▲ — lack of grounding in ordinary physical experience

Corn ■▲▼✚✪ — centeredness in crowded environments such as cities

Daisy ✚ — calm and centered amid turbulent and overwhelming situations

Golden Yarrow ▲ — setting aside anxiety/sensitivity when needing to focus

Goldenrod ▲▼✚ — centeredness in social situations

Indian Pink ▲✚ — remaining calm and centered in the midst of intense activity

Pear ■▲▼✚ — returns a sense of rhythm and proportion

Potato ✚ — feeling safe and centered

Red Clover ▲▼ — calm/centered in midst of group hysteria and panic

Rescue Remedy (Five Flower Formula) ● — centering during stress/trauma

Rosemary ▲▼✚ — inability to center in body

Tomato ■▼✚✪ — centeredness despite crowds and/or traveling

Certainty

Angelica ▲▼✚ — ability to feel presence/guidance of higher realms

Cerato ●✚ — following one's inner knowing, especially when reliant on others' advice

Fig ■▲✚ — for extreme uncertainty, unable to make up mind

Forget-Me-Not ▲✚❖ — acting with greater conviction in relationships

Goldenrod ▲▼✚ — finding one's own values despite group pressure

Larkspur ▲✚ — certainty about healing

Lemon ▲▼✚ — clarity of thought

Lettuce ■✚ — decisiveness

Morning Glory ▲▼✚ — spiritual uncertainty

Mullein ▲✚ — finding inner conviction

● BACH — ■ MASTER'S — ▲ FES — ▼ GREEN HOPE — ◆ AUSTRALIAN BUSH
❱ LIVING/AUSTRALIA — ❖ ALASKAN — ✚ PEGASUS — ✪ PERELANDRA

St. John's Wort ▲▼✚ — knowing power of one's inner light, divine protection

Scleranthus ●✚ — acting from certainty of inner knowing, decisiveness

Thistle ▼ — for inner strength to take action with confidence and certainty

Vervain ●✚ — rigid certainty about beliefs, fanaticism

Wild Oat ● — knowing one's life purpose and vocation

Challenge

Avocado ■▲▼✚ — challenges to the mind

Blackberry ■▲▼✚ — strength of will to overcome inertia, manifestation

Borage ▲▼✚ — cheerful courage in facing danger or challenge

California Wild Rose ▲✚ — overcoming tendency to retreat from life

Coconut ■ — endurance, perseverance

Echinacea ▲✚ — maintaining integrity when challenged

Elm ●✚ — confidence to meet challenging and demanding responsibilities

Gentian ●✚ — perseverance in the face of challenge

Hornbeam ● — energy/enthusiasm to meet the challenges of everyday life

Love-Lies-Bleeding ▲ — ability to endure suffering/pain, discover deeper meaning

Mountain Pride ▲✚ — courage and strength when facing overwhelming challenges

Penstemon ▲✚ — strength and courage to overcome obstacles

Red Clover ▲▼ — calm/centered during challenging circumstances with group upset

Rescue Remedy (Five Flower Formula) ● — centering during stress/trauma

Rock Rose ●✚ — self-transcending courage when facing severe/life-threatening test

Scotch Broom ▲✚ — accepting obstacles as opportunities

Sweet Chestnut ●✚ — ultimate spiritual test, subjecting soul to anguish/loneliness

Wild Rose ● — tendency to give up, apathetic in health challenge

---

● BACH — ■ MASTER'S — ▲ FES — ▼ GREEN HOPE — ◆ AUSTRALIAN BUSH
◗ LIVING/AUSTRALIA — ✦ ALASKAN — ✚ PEGASUS — ✪ PERELANDRA

Change (see Transition)

Cheerfulness

Agrimony ●✚ — false cheer which hides inner conflict from oneself and others

Borage ▲▼✚ — cheerful courage in facing danger or challenge

California Wild Rose ▲✚ — zest for living, interest in earthly affairs

Cherry ■✚ — seeing the good in everything, optimistic

Fuchsia ▲ — Appears cheerful, but hides mental torture and worry

Hornbeam ● — energy/enthusiasm to meet the challenges of everyday life

Larkspur ▲✚ — cheerfulness in leadership, especially when overly dutiful or grim

Mustard ●✚ — moving through darkness to awareness of light and inner joy

Zinnia ▲▼✚✪ — to encourage childlike humor, lightness of heart

Children

Angelica ▲▼✚ — to protect a child, instill connection with guardian angel

Aspen ● — fear of the unknown, nightmares

Baby Blue Eyes ▲▼ — lack of childlike innocence/trust, abandoned/abused by father

Beech ●✚ — conflict with siblings/peers, intolerant and judgemental

Black Cohosh ▲ — abusive, exploitative, incestuous relationships

Blackberry ■▲▼✚ — developing more interest/involvement in tasks at school/home

Buttercup ▲✚ — low self-esteem

California Wild Rose ▲✚ — poor appetite, insufficient interest in the physical world

Calla Lily ▲✚ — mixed signals about sexual identity, parents wanted child of different sex

Centaury ● — for the "pleaser," the compulsively good child

Cerato ●✚ — inquisitive/talkative but always needs confirmation

Chamomile ▲✚ — calming tension, hyperactivity, fussiness, colic, insomnia

Cherry Plum ●✚ — violent temper tantrums, food binging

● BACH — ■ MASTER'S — ▲ FES — ▼ GREEN HOPE — ◆ AUSTRALIAN BUSH
◗ LIVING/AUSTRALIA — ✤ ALASKAN — ✚ PEGASUS — ✪ PERELANDRA

Chestnut Bud ●✚ — difficulty with learning experiences, need to repeat, lag behind

Chicory ●✚ — neediness, temper tantrums, clinging, demands attention

Cleavers ▲ — throwing of tantrums and using guilt, manipulative

Clematis ●✚ — for the daydreamer, whose attention is elsewhere

Crab Apple ●▼✚ — fussy, obsessive over details, feels dirty, unclean

Dill ▲▼✪ — for travelling and nervous tension

Dogwood ▲ — emotional trauma stored in body, leading to awkwardness

Echinacea ▲✚ — severe trauma/abuse, to reclaim self-esteem and self-respect

Elm ●✚ — takes on adult responsibilities in dysfunctional/broken home

Eucalyptus ▲✚ — feels unwanted, in the way, leaves room, but afraid of being alone

Evening Primrose ▲ — to heal trauma of adoption/being unwanted

Fairy Lantern ▲ — immaturity

Fawn Lily ▲ — tendency to develop inner world, cut off from others

Gentian ●✚ — easily discouraged, upset, will quit easily

Golden Yarrow ▲ — oversensitive, encourages involvement, provides protection

Gorse ●✚ — feeling completely hopeless

Heather ●✚ — overly-talkative, especially about self

Holly ●✚ — sibling rivalry, jealousy, feels not enough love to go around

Honeysuckle ●✚ — desperately misses parents

Hornbeam ● — for those who can't get going in the morning

Impatiens ●✚ — hasty, impulsive, restless, easily frustrated

Iris ▲ — building/sustaining artistic, soulful tendencies, especially if suppressed

Larch ●✚ — self-confidence in creative expression and speech, fear of ridicule

Mallow ▲▼✚ — to develop social impulses, warmth and sharing

Manzanita ▲✚ — alienation from physical body and world, especially from birth trauma

Mariposa Lily ▲ — mother-child bonding

Mimulus ●✚ — timidity, shyness, everyday fears such as fear of the dark

---

● BACH — ■ MASTER'S — ▲ FES — ▼ GREEN HOPE — ◆ AUSTRALIAN BUSH
◗ LIVING/AUSTRALIA — ✤ ALASKAN — ✚ PEGASUS — ✪ PERELANDRA

Mustard ●✚ — unhappy, despondent, gloomy, depressed for no apparent reason

Oak ●✚ — holding on to struggle, not knowing when to let go

Olive ●✚ — restoring strength, energy after illness

Onion ▲✚ — disappointment and loss

Pecan ✚ — eases self-consciousness of being too tall, short or fat

Penstemon ▲✚ — challenges to physical development: injury, weakness, deformity

Petunia ▲✚ — calming and centering for hyperactive children

Pine ● — self-blame, hard on oneself, filled with guilt feelings

Pineapple Weed ✣ — harmony between mothers and children

Pink Monkeyflower ▲ — abuse, exploitation, shame, fear of exposure, introversion

Pink Yarrow ▲ — oversensitive in family situations, internalizes family trauma

Purple Monkeyflower ▲ — subjected to ritual abuse

Red Chestnut ●✚ — fearful of others, overprotective parents

Rescue Remedy (Five Flower Formula) ● — accidents, out of control situations

Rock Rose ●✚ — terrifying nightmares and deep-set fears

St. John's Wort ▲▼✚ — fear of the dark, sleep traumas, bedwetting

Scleranthus ●✚ — indecisiveness

Self-Heal ▲ — self-confidence and reliance, drawing on own forces to become well

Shasta Daisy ▲ — integration of emerging identity, sense of wholeness after trauma

Shooting Star ▲✚✣ — feeling alien, not belonging

Star of Bethlehem ●▼◗ — soothe effects of shock or trauma

Sunflower ▲▼✚✣ — healthy sense of self, especially when issues with father

Sweet Chestnut ●✚ — the lonely, quiet child

Tobacco ✚ — when nightmares take the form of feeling lost, unable to "get back"

Trumpet Vine ▲✚ — shyness in speech

Vervain ●✚ — high strung, hyperactive

Vine ●✚ — strong willed, the bully

Violet ▲ — painful shyness

● BACH — ■ MASTER'S — ▲ FES — ▼ GREEN HOPE — ◆ AUSTRALIAN BUSH
◗ LIVING/AUSTRALIA — ✣ ALASKAN — ✚ PEGASUS — ✪ PERELANDRA

Walnut ●✚ — for transitions: new school, new home, puberty, divorce, etc.

Water Violet ●✚ — independent with an air of superiority, aloofness

White Chestnut ● — insomnia from concerns of the day

Wild Rose ● — listless, apathetic, especially after lingering illness

Willow ●✚ — bitter, angry, resentful, unforgiving

Yarrow ▲ — for very psychic/sensitive children who need extra protection

Yerba Santa ▲✚ — gentle release of internalized trauma

Yucca ✚ — transforms anger/frustration into spiritual energy

Choice

California Wild Rose ▲✚ — accepting the challenges of life on earth

Cerato ●✚ — ability to make decisions rather than relying on others

Ixora ▼ — affirming choices about sexual boundaries and sexual relationships

Mullein ▲✚ — finding inner conviction

Pomegranate ▲▼✚ — conflict choosing between family or career

Scleranthus ●✚ — indecisiveness

Shooting Star ▲✚❖ — feeling alien, not belonging

Wild Oat ● — knowing one's life purpose

City Life/Stress

Antiseptic Bush ◗ — cleansing of negative influences in one's environment

Catnip ✚ — city dwellers with a fear of nature

Chaparral ▲✚ — cleansing the subconscious of images of violence/degradation

Corn ■▲▼✚❂ — centeredness in crowded environments such as cities

Dill ▲▼❂ — overwhelmed by the fast pace of urban life

Fawn Lily ▲ — unable to cope with stress/challenge, to needing perfection/peace

Goldenrod ▲▼✚ — attunes city dwellers to the environment

Golden Yarrow ▲ — ability to perform/create in intense environments

Indian Pink ▲✚ — remaining calm and centered in the midst of intense activity

Nicotiana ▲ — hardening due to urban stress, attraction to addictive substances

---

● BACH — ■ MASTER'S — ▲ FES — ▼ GREEN HOPE — ◆ AUSTRALIAN BUSH
◗ LIVING/AUSTRALIA — ❖ ALASKAN — ✚ PEGASUS — ❂ PERELANDRA

Oregon Grape ▲ — expecting hostility from others, mistrust and fear

Pink Fairy Orchid ◗ — stress from environmental chaos or pressure

Pink Yarrow ▲ — absorbing feelings of crowds, oversensitive

Rose-Beauty Secret ✚ — eases stress, stimulates balance in city environments

Rose - Buff Beauty ✚ — Stimulates intellect to better deal with city pressures

Sweet Pea ▲✚ — a sense of homelessness, wandering

Tiger Lily ▲✚ — aggressive behavior

Yarrow ▲ — depletion due to oversensitivity of frenetic pace of city life

Yarrow Special Formula ▲ — protection from environmental pollution/disharmony

Clairvoyance/Clairaudience/Psychic

Angel's Trumpet ▲✚ — opens clairvoyance, clairaudience

Cacao ✚ — stimulates psychic abilities

California Poppy ▲▼ — enhances psychic skills

Cape Honeysuckle ✚ — may intensify psychic abilities

Caterpillar Plant ✚ — to assimilate new psychic abilities

Chaparral ▲✚ — balanced psychic awareness

Deer's Tongue ✚ — awakens psychic gifts

Dogwood ▲ — helps release certain long-buried psychic gifts within people

Eyebright ✚ — for psychic healer/practitioner to better perceive condition of client

French Marigold ▼ — enhances clairvoyant and conventional hearing

Ginseng ✚ — opening psychic abilities

Green Rose ✚◗ — psychic balance/channeling, enhances all psychic abilities

Larkspur ▲✚ — psychic attunement and telepathy are increased

Lily of the Valley ✚ — opens psychic centers

Lobelia ✚ — psychic development

Lotus ▲✚ — stimulates creative visualization and psychic abilities

Monterey Pine ✚ — psychic clarity

Mugwort ▲✚ — enhances psychic abilities

Potato ✚ — omnidirectional clairvoyance, seeing into all dimensions

Pyrethrum ✚ — afraid of or do not understand psychic gifts

Queen Anne's Lace ▲▼✚ — to harmonize emerging psychic faculties

Rhododendron ✚ — expanding psychic abilities

Rosa Sinowilsonii ✚ — activates clairaudience

Vanilla ✚ — stimulates clairaudience

Viburnum ✚ — strengthens psychic abilities

White Hibiscus ▼ — increases psychic/sensory abilities to the higher planes of being

Clarity

Alder ❖ — translating clarity of sight into appropriate action

Apple ■▲✚ — clarity and decisiveness

Avocado ■▲▼✚ — mental focus

Banana ■▲▼✚ — ability to step back and observe

Blackberry ■▲▼✚ — inspiration, incisive, direct

Bladderwort ❖ — clarity of perception

Boronia ◆ — serenity, clarity of thought and mind

Bunchberry ❖ — mental clarity, especially during demanding situations

Bush Fuchsia ◆ — inability to balance the logical/rational with intuitive/creative

Buttercup ▲✚ — stimulates mental clarity, memory

Cacao ✚ — promotes increased mental clarity and reduces stress

Calendula ▲▼✚ — improves clarity and compassion in verbal communication

Daisy ✚ — calm and centered amid turbulent and overwhelming situations

Deerbrush ▲ — purity and clarity of motivation

Dill ▲▼✪ — confusion from the intensity of too many experiences

Forget-Me-Not ▲✚❖ — greater spaciousness and mindfulness

Horseradish ✚ — alertness and clarity of thought develop

Isopogon ◆ — retrieval of forgotten skills

Jerusalem Artichoke ✚ — stimulates intellect, stabilizes mood

Lemon ▲▼✚ — clarity of thought

Lettuce ■✚ — decisiveness

Madia ▲✚ — mental clarity and concentration

Milkweed ▲✚ — creates mental clarity in emotionally complex situations

---

● BACH — ■ MASTER'S — ▲ FES — ▼ GREEN HOPE — ◆ AUSTRALIAN BUSH
❯ LIVING/AUSTRALIA — ❖ ALASKAN — ✚ PEGASUS — ✪ PERELANDRA

Mountain Pennyroyal ▲ — need to purge negative or foreign thought forms

Paper Birch ❖ — clarity of purpose

Paw Paw ✦◆ — focus and clarity

Pear ■▲▼✚ — returns a sense of rhythm and proportion

Peppermint ▲✚ — stimulates healthy mental alertness

Pineapple ■✚ — clarity with money issues

Pink Trumpet Flower ❱ — harnessing inner strength of purpose, direct it to goals

Rosemary ▲▼✚ — develops mental clarity and sensitivity

Queen Anne's Lace ▲▼✚ — to harmonize emerging psychic faculties

Star Tulip ▲✚ — ability to contact higher realms

Twinflower ❖ — hearing and speaking from a place of clarity

White Chestnut ● — achieving mental clarity by cultivating inner quiet

White Eremophila ❱ — clarity for those engulfed in complexities/difficulties

Wild Oat ● — clarity about one's life purpose

Claustrophobia (see Fear)

Cleansing

Acacia ✚ — cleanses nadis

Antiseptic Bush ❱ — cleansing of negative influences in one's environment

Apple ■▲✚ — healthy, magnetic attitudes

Arrowhead ▼ — deep cleansing and balancing of the emotional body

Barley ✚ — strong cleanser and balancer of the meridians

Black Currant ▼ — heals cellular memory seven generations back

Blackberry ■▲▼✚ — the all purpose purifier

Bottlebrush ▼◆✚ — cleanses anxiety

California Poppy ▲▼ — facilitates emotional cleansing

Calypso Orchid ✚ — cleanses crown chakra

Cedar ✚ — cleanses etheric body

Chaparral ▲✚ — emotional cleansing, especially during dreams, cleansing subconscious

Crab Apple ●▼✚ — releasing emotional/physical impurities

Dandelion ▲▼✚❖ — cleansing/detoxifying subtle bodies for balance and well-being

Deerbrush ▲ — gentle cleanser of the heart, purifying motivation/intention

Dutchman's Breeches ✚ — etheric cleansing

Easter Lily ▲✚ — purification of sexual desires and sexual organs

Eucalyptus ▲✚ — cleanses feelings of guilt

Evening Primrose ▲ — release of toxic emotion absorbed from parents

Fireweed ▲❖✚ — cleansing outdated energy patterns from the body

Flax ✚ — powerful cleanser for meridians good with acupuncture and accupressure

Foxglove ▲❖✚ — cleansing and releasing old wounds

Golden Ear Drops ▲ — release of painful childhood memories, especially through tears

Grass of Parnassus ❖ — cleansing cellular patterns of disharmony

Holly ●✚ — releasing negative emotions, such as jealousy, envy, hostility

Indian Paintbrush ▲✚ — cleanses the heart

Jasmine ▲▼✚ — purifies the ego, cleanses the individual of negative self images

Lavender ▲✚ — cleanses meridians

Lotus ▲✚ — general cleanser and tonic for the entire system

Lungwort ✚ — cleanses one to breathe into a full experience/expression of self

Mountain Pennyroyal ▲ — clearing negative thoughts absorbed from others

Niella ▼ — cleanses and balances all chakras to state of purity

Noni ▲ — cleanses emotions to prepare women for childbearing and motherhood

Plantain ▲ — cleansing and purifying mental toxicity

Potato ✚ — cleanse and release what we no longer need to carry around

Rose Campion ✚ — cleanses and releases hurt from the heart

Sage ▲✚ — cleansing and purifying

Sagebrush ▲✚ — shedding false identity, letting go of the old, emptying

Self-Heal ▲ — overall balance/regeneration during cleansing and healing

Spanish Bayonet ▼ — thorough cleansing on the cellular level

● BACH — ■ MASTER'S — ▲ FES — ▼ GREEN HOPE — ◆ AUSTRALIAN BUSH
◗ LIVING/AUSTRALIA — ❖ ALASKAN — ✚ PEGASUS — ◯ PERELANDRA

Sweetgrass ❖ — cleansing of the etheric body

Tomato ■▼✚✪ — cleanses body and dissolves blockages

White Mullein ▼ — cleansing of the subtle bodies to a state of vibrational purity

White Nicotiana ▼ — cleansing ego habits and cravings

Wintergreen ▼✚ — cleanses illusions of false responsibility so we can be true self

Wild Rhubarb ❖ — cleansing communication channel between heart and mind

Yerba Santa ▲✚ — gentle release of internalized trauma

Closure/Completion

Bunchberry ❖ — for closure and initiating projects

Coconut ■ — endurance, perseverance

Grass of Parnassus ❖ — completion of learning cycles

Hairy Butterwort ❖ — completion of learning cycles without crisis or illness

Sitka Burnet ❖ — completion of the past on all levels

Sweetgrass ❖ — completion of healing cycles

Co-Dependence

Agrimony ●✚ — hiding true feelings, using an outer mask of cheerfulness

Almond ■▲✚ — addictive personality, sense of need, obsessive/compulsive

Apple ■▲✚ — healthy self-image, cleansing destructive emotions

Avocado ■▲▼✚ — to become "undependent," awareness of patterns

Banana ■▲▼✚ — for acting not reacting, realizing no need for credit nor blame

Black Cohosh ▲ — confronting/transforming abusive/exploitative relationships

Blackberry ■▲▼✚ — insight into symptoms/solutions, pure, constructive thinking

Bleeding Heart ▲✚ — possessive/clinging, letting go of emotional dependence

Buttercup ▲✚ — low self-esteem, lack of self-worth in relationships

Centaury ● — unhealthy need to serve or please others, accepting exploitation

---

● BACH — ■ MASTER'S — ▲ FES — ▼ GREEN HOPE — ◆ AUSTRALIAN BUSH
◗ LIVING/AUSTRALIA — ❖ ALASKAN — ✚ PEGASUS — ✪ PERELANDRA

Cerato ●✚ — inability to make decisions, overly reliant on advice of others

Cherry ■✚ — cheerfulness during setbacks, counteract addictive personalities

Chicory ●✚ — neediness, possessiveness, manipulative

Coconut ■ — endurance, perseverance

Corn ■▲▼✚◐ — break illusion of being stuck, seeing everyday as a new opportunity

Date ■ — finding fault in others instead of focusing on own issues

Elm ●✚ — securing affection by being the hero, afraid to let others down

Fairy Lantern ▲ — feigning helplessness or over-dependence

Fig ■▲✚ — accepting/honoring feeling, not too hard on oneself

Goldenrod ▲▼✚ — dependence on social approval of others

Grape ■ — finding love in self instead of expecting others to provide fulfillment

Lettuce ■✚ — clear communication of thoughts and feelings

Mariposa Lily ▲ — abandonment/insecurity from childhood which distorts present

Milkweed ▲✚ — extreme dependence

Orange ■ — hopelessness, despair, giving up, for finding what works

Peach ■▲✚ — serving others out of wholeness, not neediness

Pine ● — internalizing guilt, taking blame/responsibility for others' faults

Pineapple ■✚ — lack of confidence, for work-related issues, letting your light shine

Pink Monkeyflower ▲ — masking inner feelings, especially vulnerability

Pink Yarrow ▲ — enmeshed in others' feelings, can't identify own feelings

Quince ▲✚ — balancing polarities of power/love, receptivity/assertiveness

Raspberry ■✚ — wounds from abusive relationships, to forgive abuser, not be one

Red Chestnut ●✚ — excessive worry/concern for others, over-identification

Spinach ■ — recapture lost childhood, deal more lightly with difficult issues

Strawberry ■▲✚ — dissolve need for approval, cleanse guilt/self-blame

---

● BACH — ■ MASTER'S — ▲ FES — ▼ GREEN HOPE — ◆ AUSTRALIAN BUSH
◗ LIVING/AUSTRALIA — ❖ ALASKAN — ✚ PEGASUS — ◐ PERELANDRA

Sunflower ▲▼✚❖ — developing healthy sense of ego, feeling radiant/assertive

Tansy ▲✚ — holding back to placate family system

Tomato ■▼✚✪ — becoming loving/functional, overcoming fears, addictions

Walnut ●✚ — dysfunctional ties to family system/social standards

Willow ●✚ — seeing oneself as a victim, not taking responsibility

Commitment

Borage ▲▼✚ — difficulty making a commitment or over-committed

Bougainvillaea ▼✚ — commitment to spiritual destiny

Coconut ■ — endurance, perseverance

Evening Primrose ▲ — avoiding commitment, sexual/emotional repression

Grape ■ — loving without condition, demand or expectation

Peach Flowered Tea Tree ◆ — lack of commitment with mood swings

Plumeria ✚ — bonding, commitment to forming new communities

Pomegranate ▲▼✚ — energy and clarity to choose commitment

Pumpkin ▼✚ — procrastination

Strawberry ■▲✚ — for grounding, reliability, leave dysfunctional childhood in past

Wedding Bush ◆ — difficulty with commitment in relationships

Wild Oat ● — lack of commitment about work, goals, direction

Communication

Angel Orchid ✚ — angel communication

Angel of Protection ✚ — angel communication

Balm of Gilead ✚ — for people who care but cannot express it, stimulates dialogue

Bluebell ◆ — self-expression

Brachycome ◗ — bridging communication/mutual respect problems in relationships

Bush Gardenia ◆ — improves communication, passion

Calendula ▲▼✚ — Improves clarity and compassion in verbal communication

Carob (St. John's Bread) ✚ — group communication and interaction is enhanced

Channeling Orchid ✚ — channel, communication, angel connection, angel love

Comandra ❖ — communication with the plant kingdom

Cosmos ▲▼✚ — conveying higher thoughts in an articulate, clear way

Daffodil ▲▼✚ — deepens communication with entire self

Dandelion ▲▼✚❖ — developing body-mind communication

Deerbrush ▲ — conveying one's true intentions, purity of motivation

Deva Orchid ✚ — communication with Devas

Dogwood ▲ — grace and emotional ease in relating to others

Easter Lily Cactus ✚ — improved communication through gesture and movement

Forget-Me-Not ▲✚❖ — connection with spiritual guides

Gentian ●✚ — improves speaking ability

Golden Corydalis ❖ — communication with higher self

Grove Sandwort ❖ — communication between mother and child

Gum Plant ▲✚ — sharing truth/spiritual purpose without over-philosophizing

Hairy Butterwort ❖ — communication with sources of guidance and support

Heather ●✚ — heightens communication with learning to listen

Higher Self Orchid ✚ — Raising energy, communication, self-knowledge

Horsetail ❖✚ — communication between different levels of consciousness

Inspiration Orchid ✚ — angel communication

Lantana ✚ — communication and interrelationship with children

Larch ●✚ — self-confidence in creative expression and speech, fear of ridicule

Lettuce ■✚ — clear communication of thoughts and feelings

Moschatel ❖ — communication with the plant kingdom

Motherwort ✚ — communication with devic spirits of the water

Papyrus ✚ — all communication skills improved

Peony ▲✚ — fosters honest communication and appreciation of others

Pineapple Weed ❖ — communication between people and earth

Pink Monkeyflower ▲ — fear of expressing real feelings, fear of censure/judgement

Pretty Face ▲ — holding back from being too visible, allow one's real self to shine

---

● BACH — ■ MASTER'S — ▲ FES — ▼ GREEN HOPE — ◆ AUSTRALIAN BUSH
❱ LIVING/AUSTRALIA — ❖ ALASKAN — ✚ PEGASUS — ✪ PERELANDRA

Quaking Grass ▲✚ — ability to listen and work with others in group situations

Queen Anne's Lace ▲▼✚ — sensitizes and quickens communication skills

Scarlet Monkeyflower ▲ — to communicate true, powerful emotions

Snapdragon ▲▼✚ — tendency to be angry/argumentative in communications

Sweetgale ❖ — improving emotional communication in relationships

Tundra Rose ❖ — receiving inspiration from one's higher self

Twinflower ❖ — communication from a place of inner calm and neutrality

Trumpet Vine ▲✚ — for vitality, dynamism in verbal expression

Violet ▲ — tendency to hold back in communication, shyness

Wake Robin ✚ — charisma

Water Violet ●✚ — aloofness, not wanting to share thoughts with others

White Violet ❖ — communication with higher self

Zinnia ▲▼✚❍ — for parents with communication problems with their children

Community Life and Group Experience

Agrimony ●✚ — difficulty reading personality in group, seems happy, is tormented

Beech ●✚ — blames/criticizes others, needs to become less rigid

Blackberry ■▲▼✚ — generates ideas, but difficulty engaging will in group projects

Calendula ▲▼✚ — for poor listeners, difficulty being receptive, argumentative

California Poppy ▲▼ — easily influenced by charlatans, hustlers, gurus

California Wild Rose ▲✚ — not involved in group, wanting others to do work

Canyon Dudleya ▲ — inflating/creating emotional energy and drama

Carob (St. John's Bread) ✚ — empathy, group interaction

Elm ●✚ — takes on too much responsibility, hero complex, overwhelmed/alone

Fawn Lily ▲ — delicate, prefers to retreat in face of conflict/strife

Filaree ▲✚ — focusing on petty details/worries, destroying group enthusiasm

Golden Yarrow ▲ — ability to work in groups despite sensitivity

Goldenrod ▲▼✚ — dependence on social approval of others/status/peer pressure

Heather ●✚ — excessive need to draw attention to own problems

Holly ●✚ — jealousy and envy

Impatiens ●✚ — hasty, impulsive, restless, easily frustrated

Lady's Slipper ▲❖ — holds back from giving help/sharing talents

Larkspur ▲✚ — leadership and charisma, not feeling burdened/overdutiful

Love-Lies-Bleeding ▲ — ability to receive therapeutic support through group work

Mallow ▲▼✚ — to develop social impulses, warmth and sharing

Milkweed ▲✚ — extreme dependence

Mountain Pride ▲✚ — to take a stand, be assertive, make changes, take risks

Mullein ▲✚ — for steady flow of constructive energy in long term creative projects

Oregon Grape ▲ — expecting hostility from others, mistrust and fear

Pink Monkeyflower ▲ — fear of expressing real feelings, fear of censure/judgement

Pink Yarrow ▲ — enmeshed in others' feelings, can't identify own feelings

Purple Monkeyflower ▲ — healing coercive/exploitative religious experiences

Quaking Grass ▲✚ — ability to listen and work with others in group situations

Sage ▲✚ — seeing the larger view/long term needs, respect for elders

Shasta Daisy ▲ — bringing all parts together into a greater whole

Snapdragon ▲▼✚ — tendency to be angry/argumentative in communications

Star Thistle ▲ — difficulty giving of oneself, time or money, fear of lack

Sweet Pea ▲✚ — a sense of homelessness, wandering

Tiger Lily ▲✚ — combativeness which overrides ability to work cooperatively

Vine ●✚ — controlling others, using personal will to adversely influence

Violet ▲ — tendency to hold back for fear of losing oneself, shyness

---

● BACH — ■ MASTER'S — ▲ FES — ▼ GREEN HOPE — ◆ AUSTRALIAN BUSH
❱ LIVING/AUSTRALIA — ❖ ALASKAN — ✚ PEGASUS — ✪ PERELANDRA

Water Violet ●✚ — aloofness, not wanting to share thoughts with others

Willow ●✚ — blaming others, finding it difficult to forgive, let go

Yellow Star Tulip ▲ — to develop empathy

Company

Queensland Bottlebrush ◗ — feeling restless, tired, discomfort in company of others

Rose Coneflower ◗ — company makes one tense

Compassion

Bleeding Heart ▲✚ — learning to love another in freedom

Calendula ▲▼✚ — ability to listen and understand, especially in verbal communication

Carnation ✚ — for the pure love known as compassion

Centaury ● — misdirected compassion, overly servile

Date ■ — attunement to others' feelings, receptivity, welcoming, easy to talk to

Fawn Lily ▲ — allowing spiritual forces to flow to others

Fennel ✚ — true compassion rather than emotionalism

Gardenia ▼✚ — creates a sense of peace, caring, and compassion

Heather ●✚ — understanding others' suffering, overcoming preoccupation with self

Holly ●✚ — recognizing suffering/need of others, compassionate presence

Holly Thorn ✚ — radiant compassion, warm and loving acceptance of all

Hollyhock ▲✚ — open, compassionate heart

Lilac ▲▼✚ — the compassion of forgiveness

Love-Lies-Bleeding ▲ — going beyond personal experience to universal compassion

Mallow ▲▼✚ — to develop social impulses, warmth and sharing

Mariposa Lily ▲ — nurturing with warmth, mothering

Mesquite ✚ — amplifies compassion and warmth, great for loners

Motherwort ✚ — compassionate unconditional love

Noble Star Flower Cactus ✚ — compassion for animals, to become a vegetarian

Passion Flower ▲▼✚ — stimulates compassion

● BACH — ■ MASTER'S — ▲ FES — ▼ GREEN HOPE — ◆ AUSTRALIAN BUSH
◗ LIVING/AUSTRALIA — ❖ ALASKAN — ✚ PEGASUS — ✪ PERELANDRA

Peach ■▲✚ — concern for welfare of others, empathy, nurturance

Peony ▲✚ — supports one on the process of forgiveness and compassion

Pink Yarrow ▲ — distinguishing compassion from being overly sympathetic

Poison Oak ▲ — fear of being seen as compassionate

Pussy's Paw ✚ — greater compassion and understanding of compassion

Raspberry ■✚ — kindness, sympathy, benevolence, generosity

Rhododendron ✚ — the grace of empathy towards those in pain

Rosa Castilian ✚ — compassion in the use of power

Rough Bluebell ◆ — compassion, release of inherent love vibration, sensitivity

Saguaro ▲✚ — restores the will to live and to heal

Shasta Lily ▲✚ — compassion, nurturance, transcendence

Skullcap ✚ — to feel and know another from the other's perspective

Sunflower ▲▼✚✢ — warm, sun-like forces, radiant compassion

Water Violet ●✚ — aloofness, difficulty showing compassion

Yellow Star Tulip ▲ — to develop empathy

Competitiveness

Cowslip Orchid ◗ — for over-competitiveness

Golden Yarrow ▲ — for those shy and inherently shy and non-competitive

Holly ●✚ — competitiveness as a form of insecurity, rivalry, envy

Impatiens ●✚ — tendency to take over for others, especially feeling they are too slow

Mountain Pride ▲✚ — courage and strength to challenge adversaries

Oak ●✚ — pushing oneself hard for success, high goals that need balance/limits

Penstemon ▲✚ — inner competitiveness, meeting challenges despite setbacks

Tiger Lily ▲✚ — overly aggressive

Trillium ▲▼✚ — overcoming aggressive greed and acquisitiveness

Complaining

Blackberry ■▲▼✚ — negativity, pessimism, sarcasm, cynicism, blunt, tactless

---

● BACH — ■ MASTER'S — ▲ FES — ▼ GREEN HOPE — ◆ AUSTRALIAN BUSH
◗ LIVING/AUSTRALIA — ✢ ALASKAN — ✚ PEGASUS — ✪ PERELANDRA

Date ■ — judgemental, critical, intolerant, unaccepting, easily irritated, inhospitable

One-Sided Bottlebrush ◗ — feeling that one is unfairly carrying the load

Saguaro ▲✚ — complaining, making excuses, not feeling up to it, "I can't"

Wild Violet ◗ — fatalism and negativity about life in general

Compulsiveness

Boronia ◆ — obsessive thoughts, infatuation

Fig ■▲✚ — fanaticism

Filaree ▲✚ — obsession with details

Nasturtium ▲▼✚✪ — balance after compulsive and obsessive thoughts

Concentration and Focus

Avocado ■▲▼✚ — mental focus, remembering details

Bloodroot ▲▼✚ — enhances single point of focus, concentration

Clematis ●✚ — for the daydreamer, whose attention is elsewhere

Cosmos ▲▼✚ — inability to focus, being flooded by too much information

Filaree ▲✚ — obsession with details, losing the larger view

Honeysuckle ●✚ — being in the present rather than dwelling on the past

Indian Pink ▲✚ — remaining calm and centered in the midst of intense activity

Lettuce ■✚ — decisiveness, concentration

Lotus ▲✚ — calms mind, improves concentration

Madia ▲✚ — attention to detail, tendency to be distracted

Nasturtium ▲▼✚✪ — for those involved in intense mental concentration

Peppermint ▲✚ — stimulates healthy mental alertness

Pink Yarrow ▲ — losing focus due to emotional blurring/merging with others

Queen Anne's Lace ▲▼✚ — focus of psychic forces when confused/blurred

Rabbitbrush ▲✚ — mental flexibility and alertness, handle many different details

Rosemary ▲▼✚ — poor memory

Rubber Tree ✚ — for lack of concentration, lethargy, and spaciness

Scleranthus ●✚ — decisiveness, inner resolve

Shasta Daisy ▲ — bringing all parts together into a greater whole

W.A. Smokebrush ◗ — difficult concentration

Walnut ●✚ — focus on life goals/convictions despite social/family expectations

Wild Oat ● — clarity in life direction/vocation, choosing/committing to life goal

Yellow Boronia ◗ — can't focus, concentrate, follow a thought through

Confidence

Allamanda ✚ — inner strength

Banyan ✚ — self-confidence with learning problems, autism

Bluebell ◆ — confidence & self esteem

Borage ▲▼✚ — lack of confidence in the face of difficult circumstances

Brazil Nut ✚ — develops self-esteem and more confidence in decision making

Buttercup ▲✚ — knowing self-worth, especially with regard to vocation/lifestyle

Carrot ✚ — ambitions bloom from inner confidence

Catnip ✚ — confidence booster for athletes/city dwellers not used to being in nature

Cerato ●✚ — inability to make decisions, overly reliant on advice of others

Christ's Thorn ✚ — moving forward with optimism, peace and confidence

Dahlia ✚ — stimulates faith and confidence leading to optimism

Dog Rose ◆ — confidence, courage, belief in self, ability to embrace life more fully

Elm ●✚ — knowing one is capable of fulfilling obligations without anxiety

Evening Primrose ▲ — to find source of self confidence/worth of inner feminine

Fairy Lantern ▲ — moving forward, accepting adult responsibilities

Fig ■▲✚ — improves confidence

Garlic ▲✚ — release of nervous fears and insecurities

Golden Glory Grevillea ◗ — for those who withdraw rather than deal with criticism

Golden Yarrow ▲ — confidence despite anxiety or oversensitivity

Illawara Flame Tree ◆ — self approval, self-reliance, inner strength

Larch ●✚ — self-confidence in self-expression/public performance

Mimulus ●✚ — phobic personality, confidence to face daily challenges/fears

Mountain Pride ▲✚ — courage and strength to challenge adversity

Paper Birch ❖ — confidence from knowing purpose

Penstemon ▲✚ — strength in the face of adversity/misfortune, able to sustain/endure

Pineapple ■✚ — content with self, confidence, empowerment

Pretty Face ▲ — confidence in inner beauty, especially when concerned about appearance

Purple Enamel Orchid ◗ — practical use of energy encouraging self-confidence

Purple Monkeyflower ▲ — following spiritual guidance despite fear/repression

St. John's Wort ▲▼✚ — facing world by strength/protection of inner light

Scleranthus ●✚ — confident decision making, especially after vacillation

Self-Heal ▲ — trusting self-healing abilities

Snakevine ◗ — confidence/appreciation despite being surrounded by malice/doubt

Sunflower ▲▼✚❖ — radiant expression of individuality, positive, confident ego

Tamarack ❖ — awareness of true essence, self-confidence/understanding abilities

Trumpet Vine ▲✚ — self-confidence when speaking, greater vitality

Viburnum ✚ — insecurity, self-doubt into confidence

Yellow Dryas ❖ — confidence from knowing one's greater identity

Conflict

Agrimony ●✚ — inner torment and conflict hidden from others

Alpine Lily ▲ — conflict about one's feminine aspects

Banana ■▲▼✚ — negative attachment, loss of perspective, clouded judgement

Basil ▲✚✪ — relationship conflict, tension between sexual/spiritual

Calendula ▲▼✚ — communication problems in relationships leading to conflict

Cape Bluebell ◗ — releasing old "baggage" causing conflict in relationships

Deerbrush ▲ — feeling buffeted between the spiritual and material realms

Easter Lily ▲✚ — inner conflict between polarities of sexuality and purity

Fawn Lily ▲ — inability to cope with conflict, desire to retreat, insulate

Holly ●✚ — jealousy or envy, feeling unloved

Lady's Slipper ▲❖ — plagued by self-doubt, especially when unable to integrate calling

Mauve Melaleuca ◗ — to heal sadness/hurt which is preventing love

One-Sided Bottlebrush ◗ — feeling that one is unfairly carrying the load

Orange ■ — feeling conflicted with a sense of apathy, hopelessness or despair

Pear ■▲▼✚ — feeling thrown off balance from conflict

Periwinkle ✚ — subconscious impulses may conflict with ideals

Pomegranate ▲▼✚ — conflict between career and family, particularly in women

Prickly Wild Rose ❖ — allows heart to open in response to conflict

Purple and Red Kangaroo Paw ◗ — relationships with circular arguments of blame

Quaking Grass ▲✚ — personality conflict in group situations

Quince ▲✚ — conflict between showing strength and emotional warmth

Red Beak Orchid ◗ — caught in a conflict between desire and duties

Saguaro ▲✚ — conflict about authority or in relation to male power

Scleranthus ●✚ — inner conflict when making decisions, wavering

Self-Heal ▲ — unable to contact inner source of healing, confused about wellness

Sitka Burnet ❖ — helps one identify issues that are contributing to internal conflict

Sunflower ▲▼✚❖ — inner conflict about father image/relation to masculine self

Sweet Pea ▲✚ — conflict with others in community/family

Wild Oat ● — confusion about life purpose, career choices

● BACH — ■ MASTER'S — ▲ FES — ▼ GREEN HOPE — ◆ AUSTRALIAN BUSH
◗ LIVING/AUSTRALIA — ❖ ALASKAN — ✚ PEGASUS — ✪ PERELANDRA

Confusion

Angel's Trumpet ▲✚ — confusion over religious beliefs or mystical traditions

Birch ▲✚ — confusion of mind

Blackberry ■▲▼✚ — hampered by inertia, lethargy and mental confusion

Calla Lily ▲✚ — confusion about sexual identity

Chervil ✚ — confusion about spiritual identity

Chokecherry ✚ — confusion in relationships

Coconut ■ — confusion about sexual issues

Cosmos ▲▼✚ — for life altering decisions which often cause us fear and confusion

Daisy ✚ — calm and centered amid confusing and overwhelming situations

Dill ▲▼✪ — confusion from the intensity of too many experiences

Feverfew ▲▼ — breaking up deep seated anger, despair, worry, confusion

Foxglove ▲✤✚ — to see through perceptual constrictions to the "heart" of the matter

Mint Bush ◆ — calmness and clarity, ability to cope

Mountain Laurel ✚ — support and guidance in times of confusion and struggle

Mullein ▲✚ — indecisive and confused

Orchid ✚ — confused dreams

Passion Flower ▲▼✚ — brings stability and eliminates emotional confusion

Pennyroyal ✚ — eases mental confusion and obsession

Pineapple ■✚ — inability to choose career and stick with it

Pomegranate ▲▼✚ — confused about values of career/home, creative/procreative

Queen Anne's Lace ▲▼✚ — confusion about spiritual matters

Scleranthus ●✚ — confused when making decisions, wavering

Self-Heal ▲ — eases confusion and self-doubt

Sticky Monkeyflower ▲ — confusion about sexuality

White Chestnut ● — allows the mind to function clearly and efficiently

Wild Oat ● — confusion about life purpose, career choices

Consistency

Christmas Tree (Kanya) ◗ — for consistency of goals in a family

Daisy ✚ — easily swayed, inconsistency, indifference, "up in the clouds," fickleness

Many Headed Dryandra ◗ — consistency which brings deepening/maturing

Purple Enamel Orchid ◗ — instills consistency in achievement/energy out-put

White Eremophila ◗ — maintaining equipoise, consistency and direction in your life

Contempt

Cowslip Orchid ◗ — contempt with a sense of over-competitiveness

Holly ●✚ — contempt with feelings of jealousy or envy, feeling unloved

Contentment

Bluebell ◆ — cools, calms, brings feelings of contentment/joy

Cherry ■✚ — light-hearted, inspiration to others, seeing the good in everything

Christmas Tree (Kanya) ◗ — brings inner contentment, enjoyment of family/group

Cow Parsnip ❖ — contentment with present circumstances

Date ■ — contentment with receptivity, open-mindedness, magnetic nature

Hybrid Pink Fairy/Cowslip Orchid ◗ — inner contentment

Pineapple ■✚ — contentment with self, career fulfillment

Snakebush ◗ — fulfilling self-love

Valerian ▲✚ — promotes relaxation, contentment

Wild Rose ● — feeling soft, warm, contented, sensual, easy-going, independent

Control (Loss of)

Almond ■▲✚ — addictive personality, sense of need, obsessive/compulsive

Cherry ■✚ — emotionally out of control

Cherry Plum ●✚ — violent temper tantrums, food binging

Daisy ✚ — fear of loss of control

● BACH — ■ MASTER'S — ▲ FES — ▼ GREEN HOPE — ◆ AUSTRALIAN BUSH
◗ LIVING/AUSTRALIA — ❖ ALASKAN — ✚ PEGASUS — ✿ PERELANDRA

Dog Rose of the Wild Forces ◆ — fear, loss of control, pain with no apparent cause

Jade ▼✚ — feeling out of control, too much to do, "time crunch"

Old Maid ✚ — for men who can't control sexual urges, promiscuous

Mock Orange ✚ — fear of strong emotions, losing control

Plum ▲ — fear of insanity, loss of control, nervous breakdown, obsessive fear

Rock Rose ●✚ — deep fear, terror, panic

Scarlet Monkeyflower ▲ — fear of losing self-control by expressing true emotions

Cooperation

Holly ●✚ — ability to feel loving, inclusion of others

Larkspur ▲✚ — humorous, cooperative, caring, playful, courteous, courageous

Quaking Grass ▲✚ — personality conflict in group situations

Tiger Lily ▲✚ — overly aggressive

Trillium ▲▼✚ — overcoming aggressive greed and acquisitiveness

Coping

Broccoli ▲▼✪ — positive coping mechanisms rather than fight/flight response

Cow Parsnip ❖ — contentment with present circumstances

Dandelion ▲▼✚❖ — letting go of fear, trust in ability to cope

Jojoba ✚ — for those unable to cope with the mundane

Milkweed ▲✚ — coping independently and without escaping

Nicotiana ▲ — inability to cope with deep feelings and finer sensibilities

Old Man Banksia ◆ — ability to cope with whatever life brings

Radish ▼✚ — feeling unable to cope

Rose Coneflower ◗ — promotes inner strengthening

Waratah ◆ — tenacity, faith, adaptability, survival skills

Yellow Flag Flower ◗ — lightheartedness/calmness despite rising tension/pressure

Courage

Aspen ● — courageously facing the unknown, confronting hidden fears

Black Cohosh ▲ — courage to confront rather than shrink from abuse/threats

Black-Eyed Susan ▲▼◆ — courage to encounter dark/unknown parts of psyche

Borage ▲▼✚ — uplifting heart to face challenges

Cattail Pollen ❖ — courage to follow dictates of divine purpose

Chrysanthemum ▲✚ — courage to contemplate death

Dog Rose ◆ — confidence, courage, belief in self, ability to embrace life more fully

Evening Primrose ▲ — facing feelings of rejection/abandonment from childhood

Fawn Lily ▲ — strength not to retreat

Garlic ▲✚ — overcoming fright/nervousness through strength

Golden Yarrow ▲ — courage despite sensitivity

Green Spider Orchid ◆ — courage to face terrors and not to release information

Grey Spider Flower ◆ — faith, courage, calmness

Larch ●✚ — overcoming doubts about ability

Menzies Banksia ◗ — courage to move past pain and into new experiences

Mimulus ●✚ — courage to face daily challenges/fears

Monkshood ▲✚❖ — courage to be seen by others

Mountain Pride ▲✚ — courage and strength to challenge adversity

Mustard ●✚ — courage to confront darkness, to go through depression

Penstemon ▲✚ — strength in the face of adversity/misfortune, able to sustain/endure

Pink Monkeyflower ▲ — courage to show true feelings, overcome shame/guilt

Prickly Wild Rose ❖ — courage in the face of conflict

Rock Rose ●✚ — self-transcending courage, especially in terrifying situations

Saguaro ▲✚ — courage to trust inner wisdom and authority

Scarlet Monkeyflower ▲ — courage to face negative/powerful emotions

Thistle ▼ — for inner strength to take action with confidence and certainty

Tomato ■▼✚✿ — knowing there is no failure, invincibility

Waratah ◆ — courage, tenacity, faith, adaptability, survival skills

Yellow Dryas ❖ — courage to pioneer the way for others to follow

---

● BACH — ■ MASTER'S — ▲ FES — ▼ GREEN HOPE — ◆ AUSTRALIAN BUSH
◗ LIVING/AUSTRALIA — ❖ ALASKAN — ✚ PEGASUS — ✿ PERELANDRA

Creativity

Aloe Vera ▲▼✚ — burned out feeling, overuse of creative forces

Anthuruim ▼ — promotes the creative use of male life force energy

Blackberry ■▲▼✚ — creative poser of thought, motivation, manifestation

Blue Flag Iris ▼✚ — inspires artistic creativity

Buttercup ▲✚ — knowing the worth of creative contributions

California Poppy ▲▼ — stimulates artistic creativity

Clivia ▼ — sexual energy into concrete creative endeavors

Corn ■▲▼✚✪ — blocked creativity

Cosmos ▲▼✚ — flooding of nervous system with creative thoughts or inspiration

Dogwood ▲ — for movement artists, to feel harmony and grace

Ginger ▲▼✚ — sterility in creativity, for an artist needing inspiration and new ideas

Ginseng ✚ — clarity and release of creativity

Golden Corydalis ✤ — owning one's diverse talents and traits

Golden Yarrow ▲ — for performing artists, protection for sensitivities

Graniana Rose ▼ — breaking up blockages to creative expression

Holly Thorn ✚ — allows intimacy and the expression of our truth and creativity

Hound's Tongue ▲✚ — combining thinking/imagination, reason/reverence

Indian Paintbrush ▲✚ — vitality to creative expression

Iris ▲ — building/sustaining artistic, soulful tendencies, especially if suppressed

Larch ●✚ — spontaneous creative expression for those who stifle selves

Lettuce ■✚ — unblocked creative expression

Mullein ▲✚ — for steady flow of constructive energy in long term creative projects

Nasturtium ▲▼✚✪ — vitality, for those too intellectual

Peony ▲✚ — overcoming creative blocks

Pink Impatiens ◗ — strength of convictions, creative will

Pomegranate ▲▼✚ — conflicting creative desires, especially feminine part of self

Queen Anne's Lace ▲▼✚ — balance of psychic forces interfering with creativity

Rosa Chinensis Mutabilis ✤ — stimulates higher creative and artistic forces

Rosa Longicuspis ✤ — activates artistic and creative sensitivities

Rosemary ▲▼✚ — inner peace, wisdom and creativity

Sagebrush ▲✚ — cleanse perception, stereotypes, fixed concepts

Shasta Daisy ▲ — ability to synthesize

Snapdragon ▲▼✚ — rechanneling misdirected aggression into creative energy

Star Tulip ▲✚ — to become sensitive/receptive, a container for higher expression

Sticky Geranium ❖ — opening up new levels of creative expression

Tea Plant ✚ — enhanced creativity

Trumpet Vine ▲✚ — liveliness to verbal expression, stage presence, dramatic flair

Turkey Bush ◆ — inspired creativity, renewed artistic confidence

Wild Iris ❖ — sharing creativity freely with others

Yellow Star Tulip ▲ — artistic expression representing real feelings of others

Zinnia ▲▼✚❂ — spontaneity, childlike originality and inventiveness

Zucchini ▲▼✚❂ — releases creativity

Crisis

Angelica ▲▼✚ — for protection

Animal Emergency Care ▼ — rescue remedy for animals

Cowkicks ❱ — recovery from trauma

Emergency Care Solution ▼ — to keep system from shutting down in total shock

Emergency Essence ◆ — the Australian Bush version of Rescue Remedy

Pear ■▲▼✚ — for any troubling experience: accidents, shock, etc.

Rescue Remedy (Five Flower Formula) ● — accidents, out of control situations

Speedwell ▲ — safe and easy travel, crisis periods

Waratah ◆ — courage, tenacity, faith, adaptability, survival skills

Criticism

Beech ●✚ — blames/criticizes others, needs to become less rigid

Brachycome ❱ — criticism needing to be transformed into acceptance

---

● BACH — ■ MASTER'S — ▲ FES — ▼ GREEN HOPE — ◆ AUSTRALIAN BUSH
❱ LIVING/AUSTRALIA — ❖ ALASKAN — ✚ PEGASUS — ❂ PERELANDRA

Calendula ▲▼✚ — using sharp and cutting words, argumentative
Chicory ●✚ — fussy, bossy, critical, manipulative
Crab Apple ●▼✚ — self-criticism, obsession with own imperfections
Date ■ — judgemental, critical, intolerant
Fig ■▲✚ — difficulty with change, fanaticism, rigidity
Filaree ▲✚ — overly fastidious, picky, obsessed with the insignificant
Grape ■ — "sour grapes" attitude, cruelty
Impatiens ●✚ — hasty, impulsive, restless, easily frustrated
Pine ● — self-criticism, self-blame, guilt
Plantain-Psyllium ✚ — need to criticize others
Purple and Red Kangaroo Paw ◗ — relationships with circular arguments of blame
Rock Water ● — extremely hard on self, overly strict standards
Saguaro ▲✚ — excessive criticism of authority figures out of spirit of rebellion
Snapdragon ▲▼✚ — verbal criticism/abuse, misplaced aggression
Sphagnum Moss ✤ — inappropriate judgement and criticism
Yellow and Green Kangaroo Paw ◗ — for those frustrated by mistakes of others
Yellow Cowslip Orchid ◆ — critical, judgemental, bureaucratic

Cynicism

Baby Blue Eyes ▲▼ — mistrust, holding back, cynical detachment
Blackberry ■▲▼✚ — negativity, pessimism, sarcasm, cynicism, blunt, tactless
California Wild Rose ▲✚ — lack of interest/enthusiasm in living, detached/apathetic
Holly ●✚ — cynical hatred/mistrust
Hound's Tongue ▲✚ — cynicism from inability to contact/activate higher realms
Mountain Pride ▲✚ — transforming dissatisfaction into positive energy for change
Nicotiana ▲ — tough "macho" stance which hides/blunts deeper feelings
Oregon Grape ▲ — expecting hostility from others, mistrust and fear
Pink Monkeyflower ▲ — emotional coldness/distance as a mask
Sage ▲✚ — seeing life as ill-fated, undeserved
Star Thistle ▲ — difficulty giving of oneself, time or money, fear of lack

---

● BACH — ■ MASTER'S — ▲ FES — ▼ GREEN HOPE — ◆ AUSTRALIAN BUSH
◗ LIVING/AUSTRALIA — ✤ ALASKAN — ✚ PEGASUS — ✺ PERELANDRA

Ursinia ◗ — to retain idealism in group/family situations

Wallflower Donkey Orchid ◗ — dissolves "chips on the shoulder"

Willow ●✚ — blaming others, finding it difficult to forgive, let go

Darkness

Black Cohosh ▲ — brooding, sense of darkness with violent/destructive elements

Black-Eyed Susan ▲▼◆ — avoidance/repression of trauma/negative emotions

Blackberry ■▲▼✚ — focus on dark, unkind thoughts

Bloodroot ▲▼✚ — moving from despair/darkness to light

Chaparral ▲✚ — releases unconscious dark states

Chokecherry ✚ — clears out darkness and clarifies motivations

Golden Seal ✚ — illuminates dark corners of our consciousness

Gorse ●✚ — soul darkness: despair, hopelessness, attached to darkness/suffering

Mullein ▲✚ — not being threatened by "the dark side"

Mustard ●✚ — darkness characterized by isolation and despair

Pretty Face ▲ — inner radiance when countenance/body seems darkened/masked

St. John's Wort ▲▼✚ — fear of the dark, disturbed sleep, seasonal depression

Scotch Broom ▲✚ — feeling of impending doom

Sweet Chestnut ●✚ — for "the dark night of the soul," suicidal states

White Spider Orchid ◗ — brings love and caring to darkest corners of the world

Daydreaming

Avocado ■▲▼✚ — "out to lunch" state

Clematis ●✚ — for the daydreamer, whose attention is elsewhere, avoiding present

Corn ■▲▼✚✪ — to establish spiritual relationship with earth

Red Lily ◆ — daydreaming

Rosemary ▲▼✚ — difficult to be present in body

St. John's Wort ▲▼✚ — very active psychic life

Sundew ◆ — daydreaming, procrastinating, disconnected, spaced out, lack of focus

---

● BACH — ■ MASTER'S — ▲ FES — ▼ GREEN HOPE — ◆ AUSTRALIAN BUSH
◗ LIVING/AUSTRALIA — ✣ ALASKAN — ✚ PEGASUS — ✪ PERELANDRA

Death and Dying

Angel's Trumpet ▲✚ — spiritual surrender in dying process

Angelica ▲▼✚ — for protection/benevolence in the angelic realm

Black Cohosh ▲ — life-threatening situations with violence, murder, revenge

Black-Eyed Susan ▲▼◆ — denial/avoidance of terminal illness

Blackberry ■▲▼✚ — eases depression and fears related to death

Bleeding Heart ▲✚ — releasing attachment to those no longer with us

Borage ▲▼✚ — overcoming grief

Bush Iris ◆ — fear of death

Chrysanthemum ▲✚ — courage to contemplate death

Dandelion ▲▼✚✤ — recovery from death experience

Forget-Me-Not ▲✚✤ — to forge links with those who have died

Grape ■ — sense of abandonment after/during death/dying

Holly ●✚ — forgiving others, making peace

Love-Lies-Bleeding ▲ — profound pain/suffering

Magnolia ▲✚ — offers a different kind of midwife energy at death

Mariposa Lily ▲ — to resolve conflicts with mother/other female figures

Milkweed ▲✚ — fear of death

Mountain Pride ▲✚ — courage to fight negative thought forms about death

Pansy ▲✚ — grief from loss/death

Passion Flower ▲▼✚ — fear from dreams, association with death and religion

Penstemon ▲✚ — strength in the face of terminal illness, able to sustain/endure

Pink Yarrow ▲ — oversensitivity to thoughts/fears of others' issues with death

Purple Monkeyflower ▲ — extreme fear of dying

Radish ▼✚ — for objectivity, well-being, comfort, after a death

Red Clover ▲▼ — dealing with charged family situation during death/dying

Rescue Remedy (Five Flower Formula) ● — shock of death and dying

Rock Rose ●✚ — fear that ego will be annihilated in death

Sage ▲✚ — see life/death as a larger soul process of evolution

Sagebrush ▲✚ — to experience inner emptiness/nothingness for spiritual birth

---

● BACH — ■ MASTER'S — ▲ FES — ▼ GREEN HOPE — ◆ AUSTRALIAN BUSH
◗ LIVING/AUSTRALIA — ✤ ALASKAN — ✚ PEGASUS — ◐ PERELANDRA

St. John's Wort ▲▼✚ — fear of out of body states, anchoring awareness

Scarlet Monkeyflower ▲ — anger about death

Star of Bethlehem ●▼❱ — soothe effects of shock/trauma of learning of death

Star Tulip ▲✚ — increase receptive awareness of subtle states of consciousness

Sunflower ▲▼✚❖ — resolving conflicts with father, peace with masculine self

Sweet Chestnut ●✚ — extreme mental anguish, sense of isolation within soul

Tobacco ✚ — ability to surrender to death

Walnut ●✚ — making transitions, breaking links

Willow ●✚ — releasing bitterness and resentment, taking responsibility, forgiving

Decisiveness

Blackberry ■▲▼✚ — bringing ideals into action, stimulating forces of will

Brown Boronia ❱ — for inspiration

Cayenne ▲✚ — cutting through stagnation or indecision

Cerato ●✚ — inability to make decisions, overly reliant on advice of others

Coffee ▲✚ — helps overly analytical people make quick decisions

Fennel ✚ — indecisive, depressed, and subject to grief

Golden Waitsia ❱ — indecisive because of worry over details

Jacaranda ◆ — decisiveness, clear mindedness, quick thinking

Lettuce ■✚ — too many thoughts at once

Madia ▲✚ — clarity of purpose, ability to focus intentions

Mountain Pride ▲✚ — taking a decided public stand for one's beliefs

Mullein ▲✚ — acting on moral values, following inner guidance

Nutmeg ✚ — to draw on wisdom from past lives and one's future life

Pomegranate ▲▼✚ — conflict between career and family, particularly in women

Red Lily ◆ — vagueness, indecisiveness, daydreaming

Scleranthus ●✚ — confused when making decisions, wavering

Star of Bethlehem ●▼❱ — for creative solutions and break-through

Strawberry ■▲✚ — for grounding, reliability

Tansy ▲✚ — procrastination and lethargy

● BACH — ■ MASTER'S — ▲ FES — ▼ GREEN HOPE — ◆ AUSTRALIAN BUSH
❱ LIVING/AUSTRALIA — ❖ ALASKAN — ✚ PEGASUS — ✪ PERELANDRA

White Nymph Water Lily ◗ — using higher self to integrate and respond to life

Wild Oat ● — decisiveness about career and service to the world

Defeatism

Coconut ■ — a quitter, avoidance attitude

Kolokoltchik ◗ — fought long/hard, cannot go on, accept defeat with head bowed

Pink Impatiens ◗ — for those who give in/accept defeat when unsupported/unlucky

Purple Enamel Orchid ◗ — defeated, useless, unable to prove they can reach goal

Tomato ■▼✚✺ — knowing there is no failure, invincibility

Defensiveness

Banana ■▲▼✚ — false pride, loss of perspective, clouded judgement

Pincushion Hakea ◗ — intimidated by others' views, defensive and dogmatic

Thistle ▼ — intense defensiveness

Tomato ■▼✚✺ — defensiveness, instability

Delinquency

Macadamia ✚ — caught in contrary, delinquent behavior

Red Helmet Orchid ◆ — rebellious, problems with authority

Saguaro ▲✚ — excessive criticism of authority figures out of spirit of rebellion

Denial

Agrimony ●✚ — denial of emotional pain, hiding emotions with cheerful mask

Amaranthus ✚ — denial of spiritual self

Angel's Trumpet ▲✚ — not accepting the dying process

Angelica ▲▼✚ — not accepting reality of spiritual world/higher guidance, presence

Black-Eyed Susan ▲▼◆ — denying deep, hidden emotions, of the "shadow"

Blackberry ■▲▼✚ — denial of goodness in self and others

California Pitcher Plant ▲✚ — denial of negative emotions

● BACH — ■ MASTER'S — ▲ FES — ▼ GREEN HOPE — ◆ AUSTRALIAN BUSH
◗ LIVING/AUSTRALIA — ✣ ALASKAN — ✚ PEGASUS — ✺ PERELANDRA

California Poppy ▲▼ — not facing oneself honestly by use of drugs

Chestnut Bud ●✚ — ignoring the lessons of past experience

Chrysanthemum ▲✚ — deny aging by creating youthful appearance/holding onto fame, status, possessions

Deerbrush ▲ — denial of true motives

Dill ▲▼✪ — denial of self, of feelings

Forget-Me-Not ▲✚❖ — denying an afterlife

Fuchsia ▲ — denial or avoidance of emotional pain

Hound's Tongue ▲✚ — denial of spiritual beings/processes, intellectual materialism

Little Flannel Flower ◆ — denial of "child" in self, too serious

Milkweed ▲✚ — denying pain: using drugs, alcohol, food, sleep, etc.

Monkeyflower-Bush ✚ — issues of denial are noted with addictive states

Mullein ▲✚ — self-deception

Nicotiana ▲ — denial of real feelings, especially of the heart, use of addictive substance

Queen Anne's Lace ▲▼✚ — suppression of inner sight to avoid seeing the painful

Rock Water ● — self-denial

Rosa Nutkana ✚ — self-denial, bringing forth denied emotions

Scarlet Monkeyflower ▲ — emotional repression from fear of strong emotions

Self-Heal ▲ — denying own inner healing power

Sierra Rein Orchid ✚ — for deeply buried and denied feelings

Star Tulip ▲✚ — denial of inner guidance, of the spiritual realm

Willow ●✚ — denying responsibility, blaming others, resentment

Dependability

Oak ●✚ — to be dependable and not give up when facing obstacles

Strawberry ■▲✚ — for grounding, reliability

Dependency

Black Cohosh ▲ — caught in addictive, abusive, dependent relationships

Bleeding Heart ▲✚ — emotional co-dependence

Cerato ●✚ — inability to make decisions, overly reliant on advice of others

Dog Rose ◆ — fearful, shy, apprehensive of others, niggling fears

---

● BACH — ■ MASTER'S — ▲ FES — ▼ GREEN HOPE — ◆ AUSTRALIAN BUSH
❱ LIVING/AUSTRALIA — ❖ ALASKAN — ✚ PEGASUS — ✪ PERELANDRA

Fairy Lantern ▲ — immaturity, helplessness, neediness, childish dependency

Happy Wanderer ◗ — standing on one's own feet, to achieve with one's own strength

Lime ▼✚ — powerlessness, overdependency

Milkweed ▲✚ — extreme dependency and emotional repression

Pixie Mops ◗ — dependency/resentment cycles: becomes hard after being let down

Red Grevillia ◆ — feeling stuck, affected by criticism, reliant on others

Rosa Damascena Bifera (Damask Rose) ✚ — for addictive personality

Self-Heal ▲ — overly dependent on external help

Depression and Despair

Baby Blue Eyes ▲▼ — despair beset by cynicism, not trusting in goodness of world

Balm-Lemon ✚ — calms and represses depression

Basil ▲✚✪ — depressed from relationship conflict

Black Cohosh ▲ — depression, caught in abusive/addictive or violent lifestyle

Blackberry ■▲▼✚ — depression/fear of death

Bluebell ◆ — depression with a sense of falling apart

Borage ▲▼✚ — discouragement, grief, heavy-heartedness

California Wild Rose ▲✚ — alienation from life, not accepting difficulty/challenge

Cat's Tail ✚ — for emotional balance after depression

Chamomile ▲✚ — to stabilize the emotions, calming and soothing

Chrysanthemum ▲✚ — deep soul angst about life and death

Color Orchid ✚ — depression, sadness, creative thinking, color in life

Cowkicks ◗ — despair after physical trauma

Cucumber ▼✪ — rebalancing during depression, vital reattachment to life

Cyclamen ✚ — dispels depression, helps release ego-mind's need for separateness

Daffodil ▲▼✚ — replaces depression/low self-worth with love and trust

Dill ▲▼✪ — depression with overwhelm and oversensitivity

Elm ●✚ — despair about ability to fulfill responsibilities/expectations

Fennel ✚ — indecisive, depressed, and subject to grief

● BACH — ■ MASTER'S — ▲ FES — ▼ GREEN HOPE — ◆ AUSTRALIAN BUSH
◗ LIVING/AUSTRALIA — ✣ ALASKAN — ✚ PEGASUS — ✪ PERELANDRA

Feverfew ▲▼ — breaks up deep seated anger, despair, worry, confusion, depression

Gentian ●✚ — doubt/discouragement from setbacks, lack of faith

Gooseberry ✚ — eases depression from infertility, hysterectomy, menopause

Gorse ●✚ — soul darkness: despair, hopelessness

Green Rein Orchid ✚ — can benefit therapist, patient working with depressive states

Helleborus-Black ✚ — depression after a broken romance

Hornbeam ● — depression when facing the tasks of daily life, such as work

Horseradish ✚ — boredom, lethargy, depression, or hysteria

Indian Paintbrush ▲✚ — depression from lack of attention

Larch ●✚ — depression from lack of confidence

Love-Lies-Bleeding ▲ — profound pain/suffering

Milkweed ▲✚ — deeply depressed, can't cope, desire to obliterate consciousness

Mustard ●✚ — overwhelmed by "black cloud" for unknown reason, mood swings

Nectarine ▲✚ — depression with a need for psycho-spiritual balance

Olive ●✚ — depression stemming from physical exhaustion

Orange ■ — feeling conflicted with a sense of apathy, hopelessness or despair

Peach ■▲✚ — depression with self-involvement

Periwinkle ✚ — lifting the veil of depression

Petunia ▲✚ — spiritual courage to face blocks/denials causing depression

Pine ● — despair/anxiety about own faults and mistakes

Poke Weed ✚ — sad, depressed, and mournful

Purple Eremophila ◗ — despair over issues of the heart

Red Beak Orchid ◗ — despair/dilemma between desire and duties

Red Bud ▲✚ — depressed/distraught, contemplative of suicide

Sagebrush ▲✚ — personal devastation, hitting rock bottom

Sandalwood ✚ — fear of heights, insomnia, depression, and stress

Scotch Broom ▲✚ — feeling of impending doom

Sierra Rein Orchid ✚ — for deeply buried and denied feelings with depression

Skullcap ✚ — despair from old thought patterns/perceptions

● BACH — ■ MASTER'S — ▲ FES — ▼ GREEN HOPE — ◆ AUSTRALIAN BUSH
◗ LIVING/AUSTRALIA — ❖ ALASKAN — ✚ PEGASUS — ✪ PERELANDRA

Star Jasmine ▲ — depression from feeling overburdened

Sugar Beet ✚ — depression with "see-sawing" moodiness

Sugar Cane ✚ — sharp mood swings, lethargy, and general depression

Sweet Chestnut ●✚ — extreme mental anguish, sense of isolation within soul

Tree of Life ✚ — upliftment, eases depression

Violet Butterfly ❱ — emotionally shattered during/after relationship traumas

Water Hyacinth ▼ — lifts depression, fear, heaviness, for winter blues, lack of sun

Watermelon ▲✚ — easing of obsessive and depressed states

Wild Oat ● — despair over life's work, direction, job dissatisfaction

Wild Rose ● — apathy/resignation when faced with illness/challenge

Witch Hazel ▲✚ — winter depression

Yellow Flag Flower ❱ — depression from rising pressure and tension

Yerba Santa ▲✚ — internalized sadness, especially held in chest region, emotional pain

Ylang Ylang ✚ — calms anger, frustration, stress, depression

Zinnia ▲▼✚✪ — feeling unloved, hurt, angry, critical, bitter

Desire

Apple ■▲✚ — to integrate desires and willpower to realize goals and visions

Basil ▲✚✪ — clandestine sexual desire which undermines relationships

Blackberry ■▲▼✚ — bringing desires into manifestation

Bleeding Heart ▲✚ — possessiveness, desire to hold on to the other person

Blue Leschenaultia ❱ — rekindles the desire to give with grace and benevolence

Breadfruit ✚ — desire for pregnancy, tension in a relationship preventing pregnancy

California Pitcher Plant ▲✚ — suppression of instinctual desires (sex, hunger, etc)

California Poppy ▲▼ — craves stimulating experiences through drugs/psychic highs

Centaury ● — weak sense of personal desire, neglecting self for desire of others

Chervil ✚ — to stimulate desire to meditate

● BACH — ■ MASTER'S — ▲ FES — ▼ GREEN HOPE — ◆ AUSTRALIAN BUSH
❱ LIVING/AUSTRALIA — ✤ ALASKAN — ✚ PEGASUS — ✪ PERELANDRA

Deerbrush ▲ — unconscious desires, unclear motivations

Easter Lily ▲✚ — conflicts about sexual desire, feeling sexuality is impure

Hibiscus ▲ — repression of sexual desire

Lady's Slipper ▲❖ — lack of sexual desire due to nervous exhaustion/depletion

Manzanita ▲✚ — denial of physical desire from estrangement from physical body

Milkweed ▲✚ — cravings to dull consciousness: drugs, alcohol, excessive food

Money Plant ✚ — balance between material and spiritual desires

Pistachio ✚ — desire to curb sexual appetite, promiscuity, desire for monogamy

Quaking Grass ▲✚ — altruistic sacrifice or desires for the good of the larger group

Red Beak Orchid ◗ — despair/dilemma between desire and duties

Rock Water ● — repression of desires from strict sense of discipline, asceticism

Ruta (Rue) ▲✚ — gives energy to one's true desires and acceptance of oneself

Sagebrush ▲✚ — release of desires/cravings which hinder growth

Scleranthus ●✚ — confusion about what one wants, leading to indecision

Spice Bush ▲✚ — desire to turn fiery yang dragon into positive service

Sticky Monkeyflower ▲ — inappropriate acting out of sexual desire

Tansy ▲✚ — acting on one's desires

Trillium ▲▼✚ — greed/lust, can't overcome personal desire for common good

Walnut ●✚ — courage to follow heart despite judgement of others

Wild Oat ● — despair over life's work, direction, job dissatisfaction

Wild Rhubarb ❖ — resenting others abundance, let go of self-made limitations

Wooly Banksia ◗ — desire to pursue ideals/goals when struggle seems too much

Despondency

Bittersweet ✚ — releases grief, mourning and despondency

Cherry ■✚ — emotionally "out of control"

● BACH — ■ MASTER'S — ▲ FES — ▼ GREEN HOPE — ◆ AUSTRALIAN BUSH
◗ LIVING/AUSTRALIA — ❖ ALASKAN — ✚ PEGASUS — ✪ PERELANDRA

Hornbeam ● — despondent when facing the tasks of daily life, such as work

Kapok Bush ◆ — resignation, easily discouraged, apathy

Larch ●✚ — despondent from low self esteem

Lavender ▲✚ — despondent with a sense of failure

Mauve Melaleuca ◗ — despondent from sadness and great hurt

Milkweed ▲✚ — grief, despair, despondency, and fear of death

Oak ●✚ — allays despair or despondency

Scotch Broom ▲✚ — despondent with a feeling of impending doom

Silver Princess ◆ — aimless, despondent, lacking life direction

Destructiveness

Beech ●✚ — lashing out critically at others

Black Cohosh ▲ — attracted to destructive or violent lifestyle

Bleeding Heart ▲✚ — holding onto/manipulating others to feel wanted

Calendula ▲▼✚ — using sharp and cutting words, argumentative

Cherry ■✚ — destructive impulses

Cherry Plum ●✚ — destructive/losing control when under extreme stress

Crab Apple ●▼✚ — self-destructive attitude by obsessing over imperfections

Dogwood ▲ — abuse of self, accident prone, ungraceful

Holly ●✚ — hatred, jealousy, rivalry

Impatiens ●✚ — hasty, impulsive, restless, easily frustrated

Manzanita ▲✚ — destructiveness from lack of connection with body

Morning Glory ▲▼✚ — harmful personal habits/erratic lifestyle, drug abuse

Mustard ●✚ — self-destructive when depressed (eg. not eating or sleeping)

Pine ● — hard on oneself, emotionally self-destructive

Saguaro ▲✚ — delinquent/destructive behavior from rebellion against authority

Scarlet Monkeyflower ▲ — sudden/blind rage, extreme anger

Snapdragon ▲▼✚ — destructive tendencies, especially verbal abuse/biting sarcasm

Ursinia ◗ — out of control ego, dishonest communication

● BACH — ■ MASTER'S — ▲ FES — ▼ GREEN HOPE — ◆ AUSTRALIAN BUSH
◗ LIVING/AUSTRALIA — ✤ ALASKAN — ✚ PEGASUS — ✪ PERELANDRA

Details

Avocado ■▲▼✚ — missing details, absent-mindedness

Beech ●✚ — preoccupied with small details, faults of others, highly critical

Brussel Sprouts ✚ — to better assimilate details

Crab Apple ●▼✚ — obsession with details/faults, especially hygiene and health

Dandelion ▲▼✚✤ — difficulty in analyzing life events in its details

Filaree ▲✚ — overly fastidious, picky, obsessed with the insignificant

Golden Waitsia ◗ — for those who worry over details

Lobelia ✚ — psychic development and ability to better perceive details

Madia ▲✚ — clarity of purpose, ability to focus intentions

Rabbitbrush ▲✚ — mental flexibility and alertness, handle many different details

Rock Rose ●✚ — sense of the interaction between the big picture/tiniest details

Rosemary ▲▼✚ — tend to get stuck in petty details

Shasta Daisy ▲ — ability to synthesize many details into larger picture

Determination

Blackberry ■▲▼✚ — to overcome fear and inertia

Coconut ■ — a quitter, avoidance attitude

Flax ✚ — gives tenacity and determination to the visionary

Happy Wanderer ◗ — essence inspires a realization of self reliance/determination

Peach Flowered Tea Tree ◆ — lack of commitment with mood swings

Penstemon ▲✚ — to be able to sustain/endure

Pink Impatiens ◗ — for those who give in/accept defeat when unsupported/unlucky

Devitalization

Aloe Vera ▲▼✚ — burned out feeling, overuse of creative forces

Apple ■▲✚ — depletion of sexual creative forces

Fawn Lily ▲ — inability to draw strength from the physical world

Fringed Violet ◆ — distress, damage to aura, drained by others/situations

Garlic ▲✚ — lack of vitality due to fear, nervousness, parasitic entities

---

● BACH — ■ MASTER'S — ▲ FES — ▼ GREEN HOPE — ◆ AUSTRALIAN BUSH
◗ LIVING/AUSTRALIA — ✤ ALASKAN — ✚ PEGASUS — ✪ PERELANDRA

Hibiscus ▲ — loss of sexual responsiveness

Hornbeam ● — weariness due to lack of interest in work/daily tasks

Indian Paintbrush ▲✚ — depletion of vital forces from creative expression

Lady's Slipper ▲✿ — lack of sexual desire due to nervous exhaustion/depletion

Lavender ▲✚ — depletion from nervousness, over stimulation

Leafless Orchid ❱ — feelings of depletion for those who work in service to others

Macrocarpa ◆ — personally drained, tired, exhausted, burnt-out, low immunity

Morning Glory ▲▼✚ — low energy from destructive/abusive habits, addiction

Nasturtium ▲▼✚❂ — tendency toward dry intellectualism, lack of life force

Nicotiana ▲ — suppression of emotions leading to reduced vitality

Olive ●✚ — depletion of vitality after long illness/struggle

Peppermint ▲✚ — dull or sluggish, especially mental lethargy

Pink Yarrow ▲ — drained from absorbing negativity from others

Rosemary ▲▼✚ — lack of physical warmth and presence

Ruta (Rue) ▲✚ — easily depleted, overly absorbent of negative influences

St. John's Wort ▲▼✚ — living too much at periphery of consciousness

Sorrel ✚ — emotionally depleted in stressful situations

Sycamore ✚ — profound fatigue and exhaustion

White Yarrow ▼ — energies easily depleted, overly absorbent of negative influences

Yarrow ▲ — drained due to harsh environment or others' negative/hostile thoughts

Yarrow Special Formula ▲ — drained from environmental pollution/disharmony

Zinnia ▲▼✚❂ — over serious, feeling dull, lifeless

Discouragement

Borage ▲▼✚ — discouragement, grief, heavy-heartedness

Gentian ●✚ — doubt/discouragement from setbacks, lack of faith

Gorse ●✚ — soul darkness: despair, hopelessness

Kapok Bush ◆ — resignation, easily discouraged, apathy

● BACH — ■ MASTER'S — ▲ FES — ▼ GREEN HOPE — ◆ AUSTRALIAN BUSH
❱ LIVING/AUSTRALIA — ✿ ALASKAN — ✚ PEGASUS — ❂ PERELANDRA

Larch ●✚ — giving up after failure, lacking inner confidence to try again

Mustard ●✚ — overcome by hopelessness and helplessness

Penstemon ▲✚ — discouragement due to handicap/misfortune, need to persevere

Rhododendron ✚ — inclined to sadness, melancholy and discouragement

Scotch Broom ▲✚ — discouragement about world situation, "what's the use?"

Dishonesty

Basil ▲✚✪ — clandestine behavior

Deerbrush ▲ — mixed or conflicting motives

Fuchsia Grevillea ◗ — hypocrisy

Red Feather Flower ◗ — to rely on own energy, to recognize burdens/responsibility

Disillusionment

Gentian ●✚ — doubt/discouragement from setbacks, lack of faith

Snakebush ◗ — disillusioned from the lack of love from others

Star Tulip ▲✚ — feeling hardened, cut-off

Wallflower Donkey Orchid ◗ — dissolves "chips on the shoulder"

Dislike

Beech ●✚ — criticism of others due to high standards of perfection

Billy Goat Plum ◆ — self-disgust and dislike of the body, especially the sex organs

Buttercup ▲✚ — negation of one's vocation or lot in life

Crab Apple ●▼✚ — disgust with imperfection and impurities

Five Corners ◆ — dislike of self

Flannel Flower ◆ — dislike of being touched, lack of sensitivity — especially in males

Holly ●✚ — hatred, jealousy, rivalry

Manzanita ▲✚ — aversion to the physical body

Oregon Grape ▲ — viewing others with distrust, suspicious

Willow ●✚ — dislike of others, feeling bitter and resentful

Disorientation

Bush Fuchsia ◆ — feeling unbalanced, not trusting intuition

Clematis ●✚ — for the daydreamer, whose attention is elsewhere

Corn ■▲▼✚⊘ — confusion in crowded urban areas

Cosmos ▲▼✚ — disoriented speech which is rapid or inarticulate

Indian Pink ▲✚ — disorientation when surrounded by intense activity

Madia ▲✚ — inability to focus thoughts, distracted, scattered

Milkweed ▲✚ — blot out consciousness with drugs, accidents, illness, etc

Queen Anne's Lace ▲▼✚ — things seem foggy, blurred

Red Clover ▲▼ — hysteria, panic in group situations

Rescue Remedy (Five Flower Formula) ● — disoriented from stress/trauma

River Beauty ✣ — emotional re-orientation and recovery after shock

Rosemary ▲▼✚ — sleepiness, memory loss

Dogmatic

Goldenrod ▲▼✚ — overly philosophical and spiritually/religiously dogmatic

Hibbertia ◆ — rigid personality, fanaticism about self-improvement

Pincushion Hakea ◗ — intimidated by others' views, defensive and dogmatic

Sweet Alyssum ✚ — to transcend dogmatic religious states

Doubt

Apple ■▲✚ — overconcern with the condition of the body, hypochondria

Buttercup ▲✚ — doubting true worth or vocation

Cerato ●✚ — invalidating one's own decision-making abilities

Daffodil ▲▼✚ — depression, self doubt and low self esteem

Gorse ●✚ — lack of faith that things will work out

Larch ●✚ — uncertainty about creative expression/ability to perform

Lime ▼✚ — to ease fear and doubt

Mullein ▲✚ — doubt about direction, moral values

Penstemon ▲✚ — questioning ability to meet difficulties

Red Chestnut ●✚ — questioning ability of others to handle a crisis

Scleranthus ●✚ — confusion about what one wants, leading to indecision

Scotch Broom ▲✚ — questioning ability to meet difficulties, with a sense of doom

Self-Heal ▲ — doubt about own healing abilities

Snakevine ❱ — confidence/appreciation despite being surrounded by malice/doubt

Witch Hazel ▲✚ — holds the light of hope and promise in times of doubt/anxiety

Dreams and Sleep

Amaranthus ✚ — calms disruptive dream states

Angelica ▲▼✚ — receptivity of soul to spiritual guidance in dream life

Apple ■▲✚ — stimulates dream state

Black-Eyed Susan ▲▼◆ — need to examine disturbing or recurrent dreams

Chaparral ▲✚ — disturbed or chaotic dreams

Chokecherry ✚ — clarifies dreams

Clematis ●✚ — dreamy, sleepy disposition, integration of dream life into daily life

Coleus ✚ — for clearer and full colored dreams

Dandelion ▲▼✚✣ — answers from dreams, overcomes fretful dreams

Evening Primrose ▲ — to stimulate pre-birth/early memories through dreams

Forget-Me-Not ▲✚✣ — communication/connection with spirits in dreams/sleep

Grey Spider Flower ◆ — terror, panic, nightmares from unknown causes

Gum Plant ▲✚ — increases dream state

Hornbeam ● — desire to sleep as avoidance of daily tasks/responsibilities

Jimson Weed ✚ — stimulates dreams

Lavender ▲✚ — nervous disposition, causing difficult or unrestful sleep

Litchie ✚ — stimulates dream states

Marjoram ✚ — lucid dreaming

Milkweed ▲✚ — sleep as an escape, dependence on sedatives, sleeping pills

Morning Glory ▲▼✚ — poor dream recall, difficulty awakening

Mugwort ▲✚ — greater activity/consciousness in dreams

● BACH — ■ MASTER'S — ▲ FES — ▼ GREEN HOPE — ◆ AUSTRALIAN BUSH
❱ LIVING/AUSTRALIA — ✣ ALASKAN — ✚ PEGASUS — ✪ PERELANDRA

Orange ■ — calms highly charged emotionalism and stimulates dreams

Orchid ✚ — confused dreams

Passion Flower ▲▼✚ — fear from dreams, association with death and religion

Radish ▼✚ — stabilizes dream state

Rosa Centifolia Parvifolia ✚ — stimulates dream state

Rosa Villosa ✚ — stimulates dreams

Rosemary ▲▼✚ — sleepiness, memory loss

St. John's Wort ▲▼✚ — disturbed, fearful dreams, fear of the dark/sleep

Scarlet Pimpernel ▲ — recurring nightmares/dreams can be understood/assimilated

Snap Pea ▼✪ — clarifies purpose behind dreams and nightmares

Star Tulip ▲✚ — receptivity/awareness of dream symbolism, dream recall

White Chestnut ● — restless, fitful sleep for anxiety or mental chatter

Wintergreen ▼✚ — stimulates data from higher self/aura cleansing through dreams

Dryness

Aloe Vera ▲▼✚ — burned out feeling, overuse of creative forces

Golden Ear Drops ▲ — releasing repressed tears, contacting core emotions

Hibiscus ▲ — warm, moist soul forces in sexual expression

Indian Paintbrush ▲✚ — depletion of vital forces from creative expression

Iris ▲ — lack of flowing creative expression

Nasturtium ▲▼✚✪ — tendency toward dry intellectualism, lack of life force

Ragweed-Ambrosia ✚ — dry intellectual becomes more emotional

Trumpet Vine ▲✚ — expressing more color and soul vitality when speaking

Zinnia ▲▼✚✪ — over serious, feeling dull, lifeless

Dullness

Avocado ■▲▼✚ — missing details, absent-mindedness

Baby Blue Eyes ▲▼ — numbing of emotions due to violence/abuse in childhood

Birch ▲✚ — dulled senses

California Wild Rose ▲✚ — apathy, lack of interest in life

Cosmos ▲▼✚ — to stimulate mental clarity, especially lively, thoughtful speech

Forget-Me-Not ▲✚❖ — lack of awareness of spiritual beings/processes

Hornbeam ● — experiencing life's task as a dull duty

Hound's Tongue ▲✚ — need for more levity

Iris ▲ — lack of flowing creative expression

Madia ▲✚ — inability to focus thoughts, dull, listless

Morning Glory ▲▼✚ — dull/unresponsive in the morning, unrefreshing sleep

Peppermint ▲✚ — dull or sluggish, especially mental lethargy

Star Tulip ▲✚ — lack of awareness of spiritual realms

Yellow Star Tulip ▲ — oblivious to needs of others

Zinnia ▲▼✚✪ — over serious, feeling dull, lifeless

Dutifulness

Centaury ● — excessive obligation to the needs of others

Christmas Tree (Kanya) ◗ — duties/everyday pressure causing distance

Elm ●✚ — taking on too much responsibility, then feeling overwhelmed

Fennel ✚ — obliged to work at which you abhor routine and monotony or nature

Hornbeam ● — lack of energy for work

Larkspur ▲✚ — experiencing leadership as a burdensome duty

Mountain Pride ▲✚ — transforming dutifulness to passionate commitment

Red Beak Orchid ◗ — despair/dilemma between desire and duties

Rock Water ● — too narrow a sense of duty, leading to self-denial/rigidity

Walnut ●✚ — over dutifulness to family values/societal standards

Zinnia ▲▼✚✪ — over serious/overly dutiful, feeling dull, lifeless

Dysfunction

Breadfruit ✚ — releases tension related specifically to sexual dysfunction

Fuchsia ▲ — letting go of dysfunctional patterns

Nasturtium ▲▼✚✪ — dysfunctionally absorbing emotional energies of others

---

● BACH — ■ MASTER'S — ▲ FES — ▼ GREEN HOPE — ◆ AUSTRALIAN BUSH
◗ LIVING/AUSTRALIA — ❖ ALASKAN — ✚ PEGASUS — ✪ PERELANDRA

Pink Yarrow ▲ — dysfunctional merging with others
Quaking Grass ▲✚ — dysfunctional in group settings
Sagebrush ▲✚ — to release dysfunctional aspects of one's personality/surroundings
Spinach ■ — unhappy or dysfunctional childhood
Strawberry ■▲✚ — for leaving a dysfunctional childhood in the past

Earth Healing and Nature Awareness

Bells of Ireland ▼✚ — oneness with nature
Black Spruce ❖ — accessing eternal wisdom of nature
Bo Tree ✚ — stimulates process that leads to enlightenment
Borage ▲▼✚ — to enhance attunement to nature
California Wild Rose ▲✚ — loving and serving the earth
Catnip ✚ — confidence booster for athletes/city dwellers not used to being in nature
Chiming Bells ❖ — opens heart to loving energy of nature
Clematis ●✚ — other-worldly attitude, lack of interest in physical world
Comandra ❖ — communication with the plant kingdom
Corn ■▲▼✚✪ — feeling fully present on earth
Crab Apple ●▼✚ — tendency to see the earth as unclean, dirty, soiled
Deerbrush ▲ — impurities in the heart block attunement/sensitivity to nature
Dill ▲▼✪ — overwhelming of senses due to machines, noise, other stimuli
Echinacea ▲✚ — subjection to extreme geopathic stress in the earth
Grapefruit ▲▼✚ — to enhance attunement to nature
Green Bells of Ireland ▼❖ — opening heart/mind to energy/intelligence in nature
Hound's Tongue ▲✚ — inability to bring spiritual perception to natural world
Impatiens ●✚ — can't slow down, sense nature's time cycles/seasonal expressions
Iris ▲ — relating to natural world as source of joy and inspiration
Jade ▼✚ — to assimilate and integrate the Green energy of nature
Manzanita ▲✚ — estrangement from earthly world and physical body
Morning Glory ▲▼✚ — out of rhythm with natural cycles
Mountain Pride ▲✚ — warrior-like courage to take a stand for the earth

---

● BACH — ■ MASTER'S — ▲ FES — ▼ GREEN HOPE — ◆ AUSTRALIAN BUSH
◗ LIVING/AUSTRALIA — ❖ ALASKAN — ✚ PEGASUS — ✪ PERELANDRA

Nasturtium ▲▼✚✪ — intellectual activity which estranges one from earth

Nectarine ▲✚ — to bring one into spiritual balance with nature

Nicotiana ▲ — integration of finer etheric sensibilities of heart with earth

Northern Twayblade ❖ — awareness of spiritual consciousness of nature

Poison Oak ▲ — relating to nature through sports/other activities

Sage ▲✚ — to help harmonize with the collective consciousness of the planet

Scotch Broom ▲✚ — pessimism/despair about fate of earth

Shooting Star ▲✚❖ — unbalanced interest in the other-worldly/extraterrestrial

Shrimp Plant ✚ — attunement with nature's cycles

Sitka Spruce Pollen ❖ — supports a balance partnership with nature

Soapberry ❖ — balancing one's personal power with the power of nature

Sweet Pea ▲✚ — inability to feel rooted, lacking sense of place on earth

Tiger Lily ▲✚ — aggressive tendencies leading to exploitation of earth

Vine ●✚ — compulsion to control animals/other living beings

Yellow Star Tulip ▲ — to develop empathetic forces

Zinnia ▲▼✚✪ — childlike joy and interest in nature

Eating Disorders

Agrimony ●✚ — using food as a way of escaping or masking real feelings

Black-Eyed Susan ▲▼◆ — to face behaviors: binging, hiding/stealing food, etc

California Pitcher Plant ▲✚ — disorders with weak digestion

California Wild Rose ▲✚ — poor appetite, low vitality, lack of interest in food

Cerato ●✚ — reliant upon fad diets, nutritional plans, advice of others

Chamomile ▲✚ — tension-created abdominal disturbances, flatulence

Cherry Plum ●✚ — feeling out of control about eating, binge/purge cycles

Chestnut Bud ●✚ — eating out of habit, repetitive patterns of eating

Crab Apple ●▼✚ — fear of impurities in food or of body toxins

Dill ▲▼✪ — over stimulation in life leading to digestive disorders

Evening Primrose ▲ — prone to overeating, seldom feeling full despite quantity

Fairy Lantern ▲ — emphasis on thinness or anorexic tendencies to look childlike

Fawn Lily ▲ — lack of interest in food due to overly spiritual lifestyle

Fennel ✚ — intelligent appetite, digestion, eating disorders

Golden Yarrow ▲ — digestive problems/emotional tension from sensitivity to world

Goldenrod ▲▼✚ — overweight used to hide one's true self

Hound's Tongue ▲✚ — overweight due to overly materialistic attitude

Impatiens ●✚ — eating too fast, not chewing, savoring or enjoying food

Iris ▲ — cravings for sweets, hypoglycemic tendencies

Manzanita ▲✚ — tendency to starve body as in anorexia/bulimia

Mariposa Lily ▲ — using food as an emotional crutch or "mother" substitute

Milkweed ▲✚ — blotting out consciousness with food, eating to stupefaction

Morning Glory ▲▼✚ — addiction to junk food, erratic eating, late night binging

Nicotiana ▲ — craving for food during tobacco/substance withdrawal

Paw Paw ✚◆ — anorexia

Peppermint ▲✚ — sleepiness after eating

Pink Monkeyflower ▲ — obesity as a shield for shame

Pink Yarrow ▲ — food as a buffer for emotional oversensitivity

Pretty Face ▲ — image of fatness/thinness due to inability to find inner beauty

Rock Water ● — excessive strictness in diet

Rosemary ▲▼✚ — poor metabolic response to food, stagnant digestion

Self-Heal ▲ — being nourished/energized by what one eats

Snapdragon ▲▼✚ — crunching, biting, chewing because of misplaced libido/anger

Tansy ▲✚ — overweight because of sluggishness, lethargy

Walnut ●✚ — to break habitual ties to old eating patterns

Yarrow ▲ — body weight as a shield of protection from psychic oversensitivity

Ego

Almond ■▲✚ — immoderation, excess

● BACH — ■ MASTER'S — ▲ FES — ▼ GREEN HOPE — ◆ AUSTRALIAN BUSH
❱ LIVING/AUSTRALIA — ❖ ALASKAN — ✚ PEGASUS — ✪ PERELANDRA

Angelica ▲▼✚ — instilling greater awareness of spiritual activity, beyond mundane

Banana ■▲▼✚ — false pride

Brazil Nut ✚ — develops a healthy ego by its spiritualizing effects

Canyon Dudleya ▲ — tendency to psychic inflation

Celosia ✚ — ego, enhances ability and willingness to be seen, to stand out

Chicory ●✚ — needing and demanding personal attention

Chrysanthemum ▲✚ — attachment to ego identity

Date ■ — judgemental, critical, intolerant

Goldenrod ▲▼✚ — false social persona to gain acceptance

Grape ■ — cruelty, "sour grapes" attitude

Heart Orchid ✚ — egotism

Holly ●✚ — envy/jealousy due to emotional insecurity

Jasmine ▲▼✚ — purifies the ego

Larkspur ▲✚ — exaggerated sense of self-importance in leaders

Lotus ▲✚ — seeing oneself as spiritually advanced

Maple (Sugar) ✚ — yin/yang imbalance, lack of empathy

Oak ●✚ — inability to surrender or yield, compulsion to be the hero

Peach ■▲✚ — self-involvement, thoughtlessness

Quaking Grass ▲✚ — insensitivity to the needs of others in a group situation

Round-Leaved Sundew ❖ — releasing inappropriate ego attachment

Sagebrush ▲✚ — letting go of previously held self-image

Sitka Spruce Pollen ❖ — relinquishing inappropriate identification with ego

Sun Orchid ✚ — egotism, sun connection, balance, equalization

Sunflower ▲▼✚❖ — lack of true self-esteem expressed as bombastic egotism

Ursinia ◗ — out of control ego, dishonest communication

Vine ●✚ — overpowering the will of others with one's own will

Water Violet ●✚ — keeping one's distance from others, disdain, elitism, racism

Emergency

Angel's Trumpet ▲✚ — for wartime and natural disasters

Angelica ▲▼✚ — protection and guidance from the spiritual realm

---

● BACH — ■ MASTER'S — ▲ FES — ▼ GREEN HOPE — ◆ AUSTRALIAN BUSH
◗ LIVING/AUSTRALIA — ❖ ALASKAN — ✚ PEGASUS — ✪ PERELANDRA

Animal Emergency Care ▼ — rescue remedy for animals

Arnica ▲✚ — shock, trauma, illness, injury, surgery

Canyon Dudleya ▲ — inability to cope in emergency, hysteria, overwhelm

Chamomile ▲✚ — to calm distraught emotions

Cherry Plum ●✚ — out of control, hysterical, suicidal, destructive due to stress

Crab Apple ●▼✚ — mental/physical cleansing, for wounds and toxins

Dill ▲▼✪ — nervous overwhelm due to noise, light, air, smoke, etc.

Echinacea ▲✚ — deeply shattering experiences

Emergency Care Solution ▼ — to keep system from shutting down in total shock

Emergency Essence ◆ — the Australian Bush version of Rescue Remedy

Fireweed ▲✤✚ — maintaining physical balance during/after emergency

Golden Yarrow ▲ — ability to cope, help others despite sensitivity

Indian Pink ▲✚ — disorientation when surrounded by intense activity

Labrador Tea ✤ — moving from an unbalanced state to a centered, energized state

Lavender ▲✚ — restoring calm after nervous burnout

Love-Lies-Bleeding ▲ — wounded, bleeding, dying, extreme pain

Pear ■▲▼✚ — for any troubling experience: accidents, shock, etc.

Purple Monkeyflower ▲ — extreme fear or hysteria of a psychic/occult origin

Queen Anne's Lace ▲▼✚ — blows to the head, especially when vision is distorted

Red Clover ▲▼ — hysteria, panic in group situations

Rescue Remedy (Five Flower Formula) ● — all emergencies/first aid

River Beauty ✤ — emotional re-orientation and recovery after shock

Rock Rose ●✚ — profound fear of imminent death, destruction or annihilation

St. John's Wort ▲▼✚ — spiritual protection in injury/life threatening situations

Self-Heal ▲ — recuperation/rejuvenation

Star of Bethlehem ●▼◗ — soothing/balancing in cases of shock, extreme trauma

White Fireweed ✤ — recovery from emergency

Yarrow ▲ — protection against physical or psychic negativity

● BACH — ■ MASTER'S — ▲ FES — ▼ GREEN HOPE — ◆ AUSTRALIAN BUSH
◗ LIVING/AUSTRALIA — ✤ ALASKAN — ✚ PEGASUS — ✪ PERELANDRA

Yarrow Special Formula ▲ — drained from environmental pollution/disharmony

Empathy

Carob (St. John's Bread) ✚ — empathy, group interaction

Maple (Sugar) ✚ — empathy between healer and client improves

One-Sided Bottlebrush ◗ — focus on contribution/sensitivity to problems of others

Orange Leschenaultia ◗ — brings in touch with softness of life, empathy reemerges

Raspberry ■✚ — kindness, compassion, empathy

Red Leschenaultia ◗ — gentleness/sensitivity, reopen heart, engendering empathy

Rhododendron ✚ — the grace of empathy towards those in pain

Skullcap ✚ — empathy and compassion in the healing process

Southern Cross ◆◗ — in touch with how life is experienced by others, integrate this

Yellow Star Tulip ▲ — to develop empathetic forces

Endurance

Banksia Robur ◆ — loss of drive and enthusiasm

Coconut ■ — a quitter, avoidance attitude

Corn ■▲▼✚✪ — taking initiative, saying yes to life's challenges

Kolokoltchik ◗ — fought long/hard, cannot go on, accept defeat with head bowed

Macrocarpa ◆ — personally drained, tired, exhausted, burnt-out, low immunity

Orange ■ — the power to endure difficulties

Penstemon ▲✚ — questioning ability to meet difficulties

Pink Impatiens ◗ — for those who give in/accept defeat when unsupported/unlucky

Saguaro ▲✚ — endurance, compassion, acceptance of who and where we are

Snap Pea ▼✪ — patience and confidence, ability to move forward

Sycamore ✚ — inner reserves of strength, patience, endurance and persistence

Willow ●✚ — receptivity and resilience

● BACH — ■ MASTER'S — ▲ FES — ▼ GREEN HOPE — ◆ AUSTRALIAN BUSH
◗ LIVING/AUSTRALIA — ✿ ALASKAN — ✚ PEGASUS — ✪ PERELANDRA

Wooly Banksia ◗ — desire to pursue ideals/goals when struggle seems too much

Energy

Allamanda ✚ — inner strength

Aloe Vera ▲▼✚ — burned out feeling, overuse of creative forces

Antiseptic Bush ◗ — cleansing of negative energy

Apple ■▲✚ — energy to pick oneself up and start all over again, with enthusiasm

Arnica ▲✚ — lack of energy from past shock, trauma

Banksia Robur ◆ — loss of drive and enthusiasm

Bignonia ▼ — robust vitality, enthusiasm and joy

Blackberry ■▲▼✚ — to overcome fear and inertia

Blazing Star ✚ — awaken heart expressive energies

California Wild Rose ▲✚ — apathy, with a dull response to life

Canyon Dudleya ▲ — calming overly excited states tending toward hysteria

Cape Honeysuckle ✚ — energy, liberation

Catnip ✚ — releases stress and irrational fear

Cayenne ▲✚ — cutting through stagnation or indecision

Cherry ■✚ — enhances basic energy levels

Chestnut Bud ●✚ — stuck, repetitive cycles with no transformation/learning

Chives ▼✪ — releases power and energy

Coconut ■ — steady energy, perserverence

Corn ■▲▼✚✪ — energy, joy, enthusiasm

Dandelion ▲▼✚❖ — effortless energy and inner ease

Fireweed ▲❖✚ — grounding, cleansing old energy patterns

Forsythia ▲ — balancing energy levels

Fuchsia ▲ — emotional catharsis

Goddess Grasstree ◗ — endurance amidst difficulties, with tenderness toward all

Heart Orchid ✚ — heart energy, love, endless love

Heliconia ✚ — inspiration

Hibiscus ▲ — sexual energy in women

Higher Self Orchid ✚ — raising energy, communication, self-knowledge

Hops Bush ◗ — balancing scattered energy

● BACH — ■ MASTER'S — ▲ FES — ▼ GREEN HOPE — ◆ AUSTRALIAN BUSH
◗ LIVING/AUSTRALIA — ❖ ALASKAN — ✚ PEGASUS — ✪ PERELANDRA

Hornbeam ● — listless for no apparent reason

Indian Paintbrush ▲✚ — depletion of vital forces from creative expression

Indian Pipe ✚ — balancing flow of energy

Ixora ▼ — sexual energy

Lady's Slipper ▲✤ — nervous exhaustion and sexual depletion

Lavender ▲✚ — extreme nervous tension, difficulty relaxing

Love Orchid ✚ — heart opening, love energy, healing

Macrocarpa ◆ — personally drained, tired, exhausted, burnt-out, low immunity

Maple (Sugar) ✚ — balancing male/female energy

Morning Glory ▲▼✚ — erratic: dull in the morning, hyperactive in the evening

Nasturtium ▲▼✚✪ — lacking in vitality, dry and drained

Nicotiana ▲ — awaken heart through feelings rather than physical substances

Old China Blush Rose ▼ — grounding energy

Old Man Banksia ◆ — disheartened, weary, phlegmatic

Olive ●✚ — depletion of vitality after long illness/struggle

Orange ■ — energy, renewed interest in life

Peppermint ▲✚ — dull or sluggish, especially mental lethargy

Pink Everlasting ◗ — feel dried out and have no more to give

Pink Yarrow ▲ — absorbing too much energy from others

Pomegranate ▲▼✚ — scattered energy

Protea ✚ — peacefulness, helps to focus energy into one particular direction

Purple Enamel Orchid ◗ — consistency in achievement and energy output

Queensland Bottlebrush ◗ — healthy flow of energy, enjoy people without hesitation

Quinoa ✚ — grounding, gets people beyond power trips

Radish ▼✚ — increases life force, yang energy

Red Beak Orchid ◗ — renews energy and inspiration

Red Feather Flower ◗ — to rely on own energy, to recognize burdens/responsibility

Rescue Remedy (Five Flower Formula) ● — disturbed/traumatized energy

Rosa Castilian ✚ — greater sense of inner energy, compassion in the use of power

---

● BACH — ■ MASTER'S — ▲ FES — ▼ GREEN HOPE — ◆ AUSTRALIAN BUSH
◗ LIVING/AUSTRALIA — ✤ ALASKAN — ✚ PEGASUS — ✪ PERELANDRA

Rosa Hardii ✚ — inner awareness, light, and energy

Rosemary ▲▼✚ — lack of warmth, lowered vitality

Self-Heal ▲ — full energetic engagement

Snapdragon ▲▼✚ — lively, dynamic energy

Spider Lily ▼✚ — to transform and transfer energy

Sugar Beet ✚ — see-sawing energy and moodiness

Tansy ▲✚ — slow, lethargic, sluggish, procrastinating, avoiding involvement

Victoria Regia ✚ — explosive energy, transformation, transition

Yarrow ▲ — drained/depleted from absorbing negative thoughts of others

Yarrow Special Formula ▲ — drained from environmental pollution/disharmony

Yucca ✚ — transforms anger/frustration into spiritual energy

Enthusiasm

Blackberry ■▲▼✚ — involvement of will forces in world, physical manifestation

Bougainvillaea ▼✚ — appreciation of grace and beauty

California Wild Rose ▲✚ — increased enthusiasm for life

Cayenne ▲✚ — igniting the will, fiery action that cuts through stagnation

Cherry ■✚ — inspiration to others, optimistic, positive

Corn ■▲▼✚✪ — energy, joy, enthusiasm

Gorse ●✚ — lack of faith that things will work out

Larkspur ▲✚ — charismatic, joyful leadership

Old Man Banksia ◆ — disheartened, weary, phlegmatic

Orange ■ — energy, renewed interest in life

Spinach ■ — childlike joy

Vervain ●✚ — extreme idealism which leads to nervous tension

Zinnia ▲▼✚✪ — to encourage exuberance, joyful involvement in life

Environment

Angelica ▲▼✚ — extended awareness of environment

Antiseptic Bush ◗ — cleansing of negative influences in environment

Balga (Blackboy) ◗ — nurtures awareness of needs of the environment

---

● BACH — ■ MASTER'S — ▲ FES — ▼ GREEN HOPE — ◆ AUSTRALIAN BUSH
◗ LIVING/AUSTRALIA — ✣ ALASKAN — ✚ PEGASUS — ✪ PERELANDRA

Beech ●✚ — over-identification with environment, perfectionist leading to criticism

Blackberry ■▲▼✚ — environmental awareness

Corn ■▲▼✚✪ — discomfort in crowded environments, such as large cities

Crab Apple ●▼✚ — oversensitivity to environment, especially impurities/imperfections

Dill ▲▼✪ — nervous overwhelm due to noise, light, air, smoke, etc.

Goldenrod ▲▼✚ — attunes city dwellers to the environment

Grass of Parnassus ✤ — cleansing immediate environment

Indian Pink ▲✚ — calm and clarity in midst of intense outer activity

Iris ▲ — ability to bring beauty, artistry and sense of soul warmth

Madia ▲✚ — scattered and confused environment, inability to organize/focus

Pink Fairy Orchid ◗ — stress from environmental chaos or pressure

Pink Yarrow ▲ — over-dependence on "perfect" environment as emotional buffer

Poison Ivy ▲✚ — respect for environmental boundaries, fear of nature

Poison Oak ▲ — to learn boundaries/limits between self/nature, as well as others

Rose-Beauty Secret ✚ — eases stress, stimulates balance in city environments

Rose Coneflower ◗ — made tense by environmental distractions

Ruta (Rue) ▲✚ — extreme vulnerability to others and to the environment

Shooting Star ▲✚✤ — not feeling at home in environment, profound alienation

Star Tulip ▲✚ — increasing awareness of subtle influences/energies in environment

Sweet Pea ▲✚ — inability to feel rooted, lacking sense of place on earth

Sweetgrass ✤ — cleansing immediate environment

Yarrow ▲ — sensitivity to negativity, disharmony, pollution, noxious influences

Yarrow Special Formula ▲ — drained from environmental pollution/disharmony

Yellow Star Tulip ▲ — sensitive awareness of subtle forces in nature/living beings

---

● BACH — ■ MASTER'S — ▲ FES — ▼ GREEN HOPE — ◆ AUSTRALIAN BUSH
◗ LIVING/AUSTRALIA — ✤ ALASKAN — ✚ PEGASUS — ✪ PERELANDRA

Envy

Buttercup ▲✚ — feeling lack of self-worth, leading to envy of others
Calla Lily ▲✚ — wishing to be of the opposite sex
Goldenrod ▲▼✚ — comparing oneself with others, over-concern with social status
Grape ■ — "sour grapes" attitude
Holly ●✚ — envy/jealousy due to emotional insecurity
Honeysuckle ●✚ — feeling those of a past time had it better, nostalgia
Pretty Face ▲ — envious of the physical appearance of others
Trillium ▲▼✚ — coveting the power/possessions of others, greed

Erratic Behavior

Dogwood ▲ — accident prone, ungraceful
Impatiens ●✚ — overly impulsive or impatient behavior
Indian Pink ▲✚ — inability to remain centered, overly nervous from intensity
Morning Glory ▲▼✚ — irregular habits and life energy
Scleranthus ●✚ — confusion about what one wants, leading to indecision

Escapism

Agrimony ●✚ — escaping emotional involvement behind a mask of cheerfulness
Basil ▲✚✪ — escaping commitment by deceptive/secret sexual behavior
Birch ▲✚ — living in past/future, escapism, daydreaming
Black-Eyed Susan ▲▼◆ — fear of looking at repressed emotions
Blackberry ■▲▼✚ — living in ideas but evading manifestation
Blue Topped Cow Weed ◗ — caught in merry go round of hedonism/thrill seeking
Bunchberry ✜ — lack of focus and will
California Poppy ▲▼ — attraction to glamour, spiritual highs or drugs
California Wild Rose ▲✚ — apathy or social alienation
Canyon Dudleya ▲ — escaping by living in extreme emotions, fanatical causes
Chestnut Bud ●✚ — repeating experiences rather than confronting issues/lessons

Chrysanthemum ▲✚ — avoiding consideration of one's own mortality

Clematis ●✚ — preferring quiet fantasy and inner life

Coconut ■ — a quitter, avoidance attitude

Deerbrush ▲ — avoiding honest confrontation with self

Evening Primrose ▲ — avoiding commitment/emotional involvement

Fairy Lantern ▲ — avoiding adult responsibility

Fawn Lily ▲ — preferring monastic/reclusive lifestyle

Filaree ▲✚ — focusing on inessential/unimportant concerns which sap true purpose

Forget-Me-Not ▲✚✤ — cutting off awareness of spiritual realms

Fuchsia ▲ — hyperemotionality or psychosomatic illness

Gentian ●✚ — lack of effort due to discouragement over failure

Honeysuckle ●✚ — preferring to dwell in memory of better times

Love-Lies-Bleeding ▲ — using suffering/handicap as a crutch/excuse

Milkweed ▲✚ — blotting out consciousness with food or soporific drugs

Mimulus ●✚ — avoiding/escaping daily life due to fear, timidity

Morning Glory ▲▼✚ — escaping through drugs/stimulants

Mountain Pride ▲✚ — not risk-taking/confrontation/standing up for beliefs

Mullein ▲✚ — inability to discriminate and adhere to moral values

Nicotiana ▲ — escaping from feeling, appearing in control

Pink Monkeyflower ▲ — avoidance of intimate relationships

Poison Oak ▲ — avoidance of intimacy by projecting hostile barrier

Scarlet Monkeyflower ▲ — fear of raw emotions/powerful expressions

Scleranthus ●✚ — avoidance of making choices in life

Self-Heal ▲ — escaping responsibility for own healing

Shooting Star ▲✚✤ — not being full present for life/community

Sticky Monkeyflower ▲ — escaping vulnerability and commitment

Sundew ◆ — daydreaming, procrastinating, disconnected, spaced out, lack of focus

Sweet Pea ▲✚ — the endless wanderer and traveler

Violet ▲ — holding back from participation in group life/community affairs

Walnut ●✚ — bound by influences/standards, not able to transition to destiny

Water Violet ●✚ — keeping one's distance from others, disdain, elitism, racism

Wild Oat ● — avoiding commitment to life purpose/work goals

Excess

Almond ■▲✚ — immoderation, excess

Bush Iris ◆ — materialism, excessiveness

Dandelion ▲▼✚✤ — excessive striving

Dill ▲▼❂ — unable to cope from excessive stimulation

Hops Bush ◗ — excessive and scattered energy

Lavender ▲✚ — extreme nervous tension from excessive stimulation

Nasturtium ▲▼✚❂ — excessive intellectual activity

Peppermint ▲✚ — excessive mental activity

Philotheca ◆ — excessive generosity

Sticky Monkeyflower ▲ — sexual excess

Sunflower ▲▼✚✤ — excessive ego/vanity

Tiger Lily ▲✚ — excessive hostility, aggressiveness

Excuses

Coconut ■ — making excuses, a quitter, avoidance attitude

Saguaro ▲✚ — complaining, making excuses, not feeling up to it, "I can't"

Exhaustion and Fatigue

Aloe Vera ▲▼✚ — burned out feeling, overuse of creative forces

Alpine Mint Bush ◆ — mental and emotional exhaustion

Basil ▲✚❂ — mental fatigue

California Wild Rose ▲✚ — resistance to course of one's life

Corn ■▲▼✚❂ — sluggishness, dragging one's feet, lethargy

Echinacea ▲✚ — complete breakdown, feeling annihilated and shattered

Elm ●✚ — taking on too much responsibility, then feeling overwhelmed

Feverfew ▲▼ — nervous exhaustion, headaches

Hornbeam ● — listless for no apparent reason

Impatiens ●✚ — overly impulsive or impatient behavior, leading to exhaustion

Indian Paintbrush ▲✚ — depletion of vital forces from creative expression

● BACH — ■ MASTER'S — ▲ FES — ▼ GREEN HOPE — ◆ AUSTRALIAN BUSH
◗ LIVING/AUSTRALIA — ✤ ALASKAN — ✚ PEGASUS — ❂ PERELANDRA

Lady's Slipper ▲❖ — nervous exhaustion and sexual depletion

Lavender ▲✚ — nervous burnout

Macrocarpa ◆ — personally drained, tired, exhausted, burnt-out, low immunity

Morning Glory ▲▼✚ — reliance on stimulants, difficulty rising in the morning

Nasturtium ▲▼✚✪ — hyperactivity of mental forces leading to extreme fatigue

Oak ●✚ — pushing oneself even when exhausted

Olive ●✚ — depletion of vitality after long illness/struggle

Penstemon ▲✚ — strength to move through exhaustion

Peppermint ▲✚ — dull or sluggish, especially mental lethargy

Self-Heal ▲ — inability to contact inner healing forces

Sycamore ✚ — profound fatigue and exhaustion

Valerian ▲✚ — exhaustion, disturbed sleep, tension, stress

Vervain ●✚ — extreme idealism which leads to nervous tension/exhaustion

White Chestnut ● — worries which drain energies and deprive one of sleep

Wild Rose ● — apathy/resignation when faced with illness/challenge

Yerba Santa ▲✚ — deep melancholia, feelings of wasting away, deterioration

Exploitation (see Abuse)

Failure

Buttercup ▲✚ — feeling vocation/contribution does not count

Elm ●✚ — feeling one is a failure or letting others down

Gentian ●✚ — undue doubt/discouragement from setback or failure

Larch ●✚ — fear/anticipation of failure due to poor self-image

Lettuce ■✚ — indecisive, emotional congestion

Oak ●✚ — resistance to failure, attachment to hero role

Penstemon ▲✚ — overcoming failure with increased strength/determination

Tomato ■▼✚✪ — knowing there is no failure

Wooly Banksia ◗ — able to face new goals without fear of inevitable failure

---

● BACH — ■ MASTER'S — ▲ FES — ▼ GREEN HOPE — ◆ AUSTRALIAN BUSH
◗ LIVING/AUSTRALIA — ❖ ALASKAN — ✚ PEGASUS — ✪ PERELANDRA

Faith

Angelica ▲▼✚ — trusting in higher guidance

Aspen ● — courageously facing the unknown

Baby Blue Eyes ▲▼ — trusting in life, especially if jaded

Borage ▲▼✚ — faith that life will work out

Brazil Nut ✚ — eases vacillation, especially in one's faith

California Wild Rose ▲✚ — trust in the value and meaning of life

Cherry Plum ●✚ — sensing/trusting higher forces, despite intense stress

Dahlia ✚ — stimulates faith and confidence leading to optimism

Forget-Me-Not ▲✚✣ — knowing there is life beyond physical realm

French Marigold ▼ — inner light, hope, faith and good cheer

Grey Spider Flower ◆ — faith and courage

Maltese Cross ▼ — to cross the bridge from fear into faith

Mimulus ●✚ — faith one can meet challenges of everyday life

Old China Blush Rose ▼ — faith in ability to make changes to move forward

Oregon Grape ▲ — accepting goodwill of others

Sage ▲✚ — faith in destiny

Scotch Broom ▲✚ — seeing societal/global problems as opportunities for growth

Self-Heal ▲ — faith in ability to heal self

Sweet Chestnut ●✚ — restoring faith when stretched beyond limits

Thistle ▼ — a lack of trust or faith in their spiritual connection

Waratah ◆ — courage, tenacity, faith, adaptability, survival skills

Wheat ✚ — stimulates faith and confidence leading to optimism

Wisteria ◆ — inner faith

Witch Hazel ▲✚ — holds the light of hope and promise in times of doubt/anxiety

False Persona

Agrimony ●✚ — hiding true feelings behind a mask of cheerfulness

Calla Lily ▲✚ — false identification with opposite sex

Canyon Dudleya ▲ — attachment to overly spiritual/psychic persona

Chrysanthemum ▲✚ — attachment to wealth, social standing from fear of death

Fairy Lantern ▲ — presenting a demeanor of helplessness, dependency

Fuchsia ▲ — hides mental torture and worry behind a carefree mask

---

Goldenrod ▲▼✚ — false persona in group situations to win social approval

Lotus ▲✚ — spiritual egotism

Nicotiana ▲ — macho personality, numbing/suppressing real feelings

Peony ▲✚ — false persona or mask

Pink Monkeyflower ▲ — fear of exposing true feelings

Pretty Face ▲ — obsessive personal grooming

Purple Monkeyflower ▲ — false religious identity/allegiance from fear of censure

Rabbit Orchid ◗ — to not rely on external images and masks

Sagebrush ▲✚ — false or dysfunctional self-image

Sunflower ▲▼✚✤ — excessive ego/vanity

Family Issues

Balga (Blackboy) ◗ — family spirit

Bluebell ◆ — need for confidence in family competitiveness

Boab ◆ — release of abusive thought patterns from family

Catspaw ◗ — to express hurt feelings, bringing reality to obligatory relationships

Christmas Tree (Kanya) ◗ — to fulfill family responsibilities

Cinquefoil ✚ — deeper attunement to biological family

Curry Leaf Tree ✚ — synergy in family relationships

Dagger Hakea ◆ — resentment, bitterness toward family

Eucalyptus ▲✚ — family disagreements, seeing the other side

Fairy Lantern ▲ — childlike dependency from overprotective parents

Goldenrod ▲▼✚ — easily influenced by family ties

Many Headed Dryandra ◗ — desire to run from family responsibilities

Plumeria ✚ — for family bonding

Pomegranate ▲▼✚ — conflict between career and family, particularly in women

Red Beak Orchid ◗ — adolescence/mid-life dilemmas about duties and family ties

Red Clover ▲▼ — helpful during emotionally charged family situations

Red Feather Flower ◗ — to recognize family burdens/responsibility

Red Leschenaultia ◗ — harshness/brittle attitudes stopping love/joy/closeness

Sunflower ▲▼✚✤ — father issues

● BACH — ■ MASTER'S — ▲ FES — ▼ GREEN HOPE — ◆ AUSTRALIAN BUSH
◗ LIVING/AUSTRALIA — ✤ ALASKAN — ✚ PEGASUS — ◎ PERELANDRA

Sweet Pea ▲✚ — the endless wanderer and traveler from moving frequently as child

Tansy ▲✚ — slow, lethargic, sluggish, procrastinating from childhood trauma

Ursinia ❱ — integration and wisdom in working with family

Walnut ●✚ — overly influenced by family beliefs/values

Yellow Dryas ❖ — remaining connected to family during growth/transition

Fanaticism

California Poppy ▲▼ — susceptibility to fanatical or extreme causes/movements

Canyon Dudleya ▲ — stirred up or extreme emotions, tending to hysteria

Fig ■▲✚ — difficulty with change, fanaticism, rigidity

Hibbertia ◆ — rigid personality, fanaticism about self-improvement

Vervain ●✚ — trying to convert others to one's beliefs, intense enthusiasm

Vine ●✚ — imposing one's will on others

Father and Fathering

Baby Blue Eyes ▲▼ — disturbed relationship to father

Bed Straw ▲✚ — father image problems

Chrysanthemum ▲✚ — desire for wealth/status/power which overshadows values

Elm ●✚ — overwhelmed/despondent from fatherhood responsibilities

Fairy Lantern ▲ — avoiding fatherly responsibilities from emotional immaturity, jealous of wife's motherly attention to children, wants for self

Fawn Lily ▲ — aloof from family — preoccupied with other worldly spiritual values

Jacob's Ladder ❖✚ — history of incest with father

Larch ●✚ — lack of confidence in father role

Pine ● — internalizing guilt/self-blame from strict/harsh father

Pink Monkeyflower ▲ — emotionally unavailable from childhood abuse

Quince ▲✚ — vacillating between strictness and permissiveness

Red Helmet Orchid ◆ — helps father/child bonding, sensitivity, respect

Sage ▲✚ — realizing elder wisdom in father/male figures, learn from father role

Saguaro ▲✚ — alienated from being father from conflict/abuse with father

Scarlet Monkeyflower ▲ — episodes of rage/power battles with child, feeling powerless from unresolved anger/power issues

Scarlet Pimpernel ▲ — for men, difficulty with father

Sunflower ▲▼✚❖ — general remedy for healing issues with father

Sweet Pea ▲✚ — lack of family commitment, fathers who travel often, uproot

Vine ●✚ — exerting harsh/extreme control over children

Zinnia ▲▼✚✪ — to contacting inner child to counterbalance avoidance of children

Fear

Almond ■▲✚ — fear of growing old

Angelica ▲▼✚ — overcoming fear by connecting to higher realms

Asparagus ✚ — release of hidden fears

Aspen ● — vague anxieties, unconscious fears

Blackberry ■▲▼✚ — fear of death

Black Cohosh ▲ — fear of threatening/violent/abusive relationships

Black-Eyed Susan ▲▼◆ — fear of powerful emotions

Bluebell ◆ — fear of lack

Bog Rosemary ❖ — release of fear through trust

Bougainvillaea ▼✚ — when anxiety, fear or mediocrity swamps us

Bush Iris ◆ — fear of death

Calendula ▲▼✚ — releasing fear

California Pitcher Plant ▲✚ — fear of the instinctual aspects of the self

Catnip ✚ — irrational fears

Cherry Plum ●✚ — fear of losing control/becoming destructive

Chrysanthemum ▲✚ — fear of death and dying

Cotton ▲▼✚ — release of burden of fear

Cucumber ▼✪ — release of fear

Daffodil ▲▼✚ — fear of religious sects

Dampiera ◗ — fear of letting go and letting life flow

Date Palm ▼✚ — fear of aging

Dill ▲▼✪ — fear of aging, dying

Dog Rose ◆ — fearful, shy, apprehensive of others, niggling fears

Dog Rose of the Wild Forces ◆ — fear, loss of control, pain with no apparent cause

Echinacea ▲✚ — fear of change

Emergency Care Solution ▼ — the Green Hope version of Rescue Remedy

Emergency Essence ◆ — the Australian Bush version of Rescue Remedy

Fairy Lantern ▲ — fear of growing up, of adult identity

Fawn Lily ▲ — deep soul fear of contamination by physical world

Fig ■▲✚ — fear of unknown origin

Filaree ▲✚ — petty worries/anxieties, especially with compulsive behavior

Forget-Me-Not ▲✚❖ — release of fear and pain held deep in the subconscious

Garlic ▲✚ — nervous fear, weakness, devitalization, stage fright

Golden Yarrow ▲ — performance anxiety

Green Bog Orchid ❖ — release of pain and fear held deep in the heart

Green Spider Orchid ◆ — nightmares, phobias

Helleborus-Black ✚ — fear of dying

Holly ●✚ — fear that others will receive more love and attention

Holly Thorn ✚ — fear of rejection

Illawara FlameTree ◆ — fear of responsibility

Larch ●✚ — fearful anticipation of others' judgement, fear of failure

Mallow ▲▼✚ — fear of aging

Maltese Cross ▼ — to cross the bridge from fear into faith

Menzies Banksia ◗ — fear of being emotionally hurt

Mignonette ▼ — fear of the unknown

Milkweed ▲✚ — fear of death

Mimulus ●✚ — worries of daily life, specific/known fears, timidity

Money Plant ✚ — fear of success

Monkshood ▲✚❖ — relating to the world with fearlessness

Mountain Pride ▲✚ — fear of adverse forces of our time

Mulla Mulla ◆ — fear of fire

Mutabalis Rose ▼ — reduction of fear

Orange ■ — fear of unknown origin

Oregon Grape ▲ — paranoia, expecting hostility

Paw Paw ✚◆ — fear of food

● BACH — ■ MASTER'S — ▲ FES — ▼ GREEN HOPE — ◆ AUSTRALIAN BUSH
◗ LIVING/AUSTRALIA — ❖ ALASKAN — ✚ PEGASUS — ✪ PERELANDRA

Peony ▲✚ — fear of intimacy

Pink Monkeyflower ▲ — fear of expressing true feelings, of being exposed

Poison Oak ▲ — fear of intimate contact, of being vulnerable

Red Chestnut ●✚ — concern/worry for others, excessive fear of others' safety

Red Clover ▲▼ — fear of own emotions

Rescue Remedy (Five Flower Formula) ● — extreme fears, no other remedy found

Ribbon Pea ❖ — to rise above fear/foreboding that prevents initiatives

Rock Rose ●✚ — profound fear of imminent death, destruction or annihilation

Rosa California ✚ — phobias associated with small, closed places

St. John's Wort ▲▼✚ — fear during dreams, out of body traumas

Scarlet Monkeyflower ▲ — fear of powerful emotions, especially anger

Scarlet Pimpernel ▲ — fear of the world

Soapberry ❖ — fear of nature

Star Thistle ▲ — fear of lack, leading to stinginess

Sticky Monkeyflower ▲ — conflict/fear of intimacy, of being vulnerable

Strawberry ■▲✚ — fear of aging

Summer Squash ▼✪ — daily fears, phobias

Sweet Flag ✚ — extreme anxiety, stress, fear

Sweet Pea ▲✚ — fear of social commitment in family/community

Tomato ■▼✚✪ — fear, weakness, nightmares, withdrawal

Tundra Rose ❖ — overcoming fear of death

Violet ▲ — fear of losing individuality in group, tendency to shyness/retreat

Wisteria ◆ — fear stemming from sexual abuse

Yucca ✚ — fear of leaving home town

Feminine Consciousness

Alpine Lily ▲ — conflict about one's feminine aspects

Baby Blue Eyes ▲▼ — distrust/hostility toward men: wounded by father

Bleeding Heart ▲✚ — tendency toward co-dependent relationships

Buttercup ▲✚ — low self-esteem, seeing women's roles as inferior

Calla Lily ▲✚ — pressure/desire to be male although born female

Canyon Dudleya ▲ — hysteria/out-of-body states

● BACH — ■ MASTER'S — ▲ FES — ▼ GREEN HOPE — ◆ AUSTRALIAN BUSH
❱ LIVING/AUSTRALIA — ❖ ALASKAN — ✚ PEGASUS — ✪ PERELANDRA

Corn ■▲▼✚✪ — archetype of earth mother

Easter Lily ▲✚ — difficulty integrating female sexual identity

Evening Primrose ▲ — wounded female identity issues with mother

Fairy Lantern ▲ — desire to remain a little girl, helpless, dependent

Fawn Lily ▲ — for the "ice princess"

Goddess Grasstree ◗ — maturing of the female principle from within

Green Fairy Orchid ✤ — balancing male and female energies in the heart

Hibiscus ▲ — sexual energy in women

Iris ▲ — ability to bring beauty, artistry and sense of soul warmth

Lady's Slipper ▲✤ — nervous depletion interfering with sexual vitality

Love-Lies-Bleeding ▲ — intense physical suffering/mental anguish with metrorrhagia

Macrozamia ◗ — balance to all aspects of male/female

Mariposa Lily ▲ — receptive to human love, maternal nurturing, ability to mother

Mugwort ▲✚ — enhancing/balancing female qualities

Paper Birch ✤ — greater awareness of the feminine

Pink Monkeyflower ▲ — feelings of extreme vulnerability/shame from abuse

Pink Yarrow ▲ — overly feminine merging

Poison Oak ▲ — fear of being engulfed in feminine, fear of intimacy

Pomegranate ▲▼✚ — conflict between career and family

Pretty Face ▲ — obsessive personal grooming

Quince ▲✚ — developing strength of live, feminine power

Saguaro ▲✚ — alienation toward men

Sitka Spruce Pollen ✤ — blending power of masculine and feminine

Snapdragon ▲▼✚ — repressed libido due to female stereotype

Star Tulip ▲✚ — opening feminine aspect of self to higher worlds

Sunflower ▲▼✚✤ — integrating positive masculine animus

Tiger Lily ▲✚ — balancing masculine assertiveness

W.A. Smokebrush ◗ — for vague fears/anxieties

Willow ●✚ — "victim" consciousness, resentment, blaming

Yellow Star Tulip ▲ — developing feminine forces of listening/attunement

---

● BACH — ■ MASTER'S — ▲ FES — ▼ GREEN HOPE — ◆ AUSTRALIAN BUSH
◗ LIVING/AUSTRALIA — ✤ ALASKAN — ✚ PEGASUS — ✪ PERELANDRA

Flexibility

Dandelion ▲▼✚❖ — release of emotional blockages causing strictness

Dogwood ▲ — harsh, cold, rigid emotions and bodily movements

Fig ■▲✚ — difficulty with change, fanaticism, rigidity

Lamb's Quarters ❖ — mental flexibility

Oak ●✚ — more flexibility in struggle, knowing limits, when to let go

Quaking Grass ▲✚ — flexibility in group situations, seeing all sides

Rabbitbrush ▲✚ — mental flexibility and alertness, handle many different details

Rock Water ● — developing a flowing attitude toward life

Wild Rhubarb ❖ — letting go of self-made limitations

Willow ●✚ — accepting, forgiving, letting go of resentment

Vine ●✚ — tolerance for the individuality of others

Focus

Avocado ■▲▼✚ — missing details, absent-mindedness

Bed Straw ▲✚ — cannot study or focus on their career

Blackberry ■▲▼✚ — mental clarity

Bloodroot ▲▼✚ — single point of focus, concentration, and meditation

Blue China Orchid ◗ — to strengthen will and take back control of self

Bunchberry ❖ — lack of focus and will

Carnation ✚ — inability to focus on present

Corn ■▲▼✚✪ — focusing when facing new life directions

Correa ◗ — from inner acceptance - to focus - to success

Cosmos ▲▼✚ — to stimulate mental clarity, especially lively, thoughtful speech

Daisy ✚ — calm and centered amid confusing and overwhelming situations

Feverfew ▲▼ — ability to focus on mental level

Golden Corydalis ❖ — focus for the growth of the personality

Honeysuckle ●✚ — helps to focus the mind on the present

Hops Bush ◗ — excessive and scattered energy

Icelandic Poppy ❖ — spiritual focus

Indian Pink ▲✚ — focus in midst of intense outer activity

Madia ▲✚ — scattered and confused environment, inability to organize/focus

One-Sided Bottlebrush ◗ — essence of awareness and balance of focus

---

● BACH — ■ MASTER'S — ▲ FES — ▼ GREEN HOPE — ◆ AUSTRALIAN BUSH
◗ LIVING/AUSTRALIA — ❖ ALASKAN — ✚ PEGASUS — ✪ PERELANDRA

Paw Paw ✚◆ — focus and clarity

Peppermint ▲✚ — dull or sluggish, especially mental lethargy

Pink Trumpet Flower ◗ — harnessing inner strength of purpose, direct it to goals

Red Lily ◆ — grounded, focused, living in the present

Rosa Kamtchatica ✚ — ability to focus will and perseverance

Shasta Daisy ▲ — ability to synthesize many details into larger picture

Sticky Geranium ❖ — focused release of creative energy

Sundew ◆ — lack of focus

Wild Iris ❖ — focused release of creative energy

Wild Oat ● — chronic lack of focus

Yellow Boronia ◗ — can't focus, concentrate, follow a thought through

Forgetfulness

Avocado ■▲▼✚ — missing details, absent-mindedness

Rosemary ▲▼✚ — disoriented, forgetfulness, drowsiness

Forgiveness

Acacia ✚ — forgiving yourself and giving to yourself

Baby Blue Eyes ▲▼ — heal cynicism through forgiveness/acceptance of past trauma

Beech ●✚ — forgiving faults in others

Black Kangaroo Paw ◗ — forgiveness/love, helpful in break-ups, grief/anger cycles

Blue Elf Viola ❖ — forgiveness through the release of anger

Calla Lily ▲✚ — forgiveness, allows a greater and deeper expression of love

Clarksia ✚ — the energies of forgiveness

Dagger Hakea ◆ — forgiveness, open expression of feelings

Dampiera ◗ — letting go and letting life flow

Golden Ear Drops ▲ — letting go/healing childhood trauma

Hawthorne ✚ — trust, forgiveness, helps to cleanse the heart of negativity

Holly ●✚ — ability to drop feelings of separateness

Hyssop ▲▼✚ — releasing feelings of guilt with self-forgiveness

Lilac ▲▼✚ — the compassion of forgiveness

Mariposa Lily ▲ — making peace with childhood, especially with mother

Mountain Devil ◆ — unconditional love, forgiveness, happiness, inner peace

Mountain Wormwood ✤ — forgiveness of old wounds in relationships

Old Maid ✚ — acceptance/forgiveness of one's parents

Petunia St. Germain ▼ — forgiveness and transmutation of all negativity

Peony ▲✚ — forgiveness and compassion

Pine ● — self-forgiveness

Pink Mulla Mulla ◆ — forgiveness, trusting, opening up

Pixie Mops ◗ — forgiveness so one does not become like those resented

Prickly Poppy ✚ — forgiveness of past life actions and those of others

Raspberry ■✚ — "turning the other cheek," releasing old wounds, forgiveness

Rosa Horrida ✚ — forgiveness for the human condition

Sage ▲✚ — making peace with life, especially as part of aging process

Water Violet ●✚ — self-forgiveness

Willow ●✚ — accepting, forgiving, letting go of resentment

Freedom

Bird of Paradise ✚ — freedom, understanding of flight/movement and territoriality

Bleeding Heart ▲✚ — respecting the freedom of the other in relationships

Calla Lily ▲✚ — returning a sense of joy and freedom

Centaury ● — freedom from unwarranted domination by others

Chestnut Bud ●✚ — freedom from needless repetition in life experience

Fairy Lantern ▲ — confusion of freedom/responsibility, childishness/escapism

Freesia ▼ — inner freedom

Fuchsia Grevillea ◗ — freedom of truthfully showing one's true thoughts/intentions

Iris ▲ — transcending a sense of limitation or weight

Magnolia ▲✚ — increases sense of freedom and relaxation

Morning Glory ▲▼✚ — freedom from erratic/devitalizing habits/addictions

Mountain Wormwood ✤ — freedom through forgiveness

Pine ● — freedom from guilt and blame

● BACH — ■ MASTER'S — ▲ FES — ▼ GREEN HOPE — ◆ AUSTRALIAN BUSH
◗ LIVING/AUSTRALIA — ✤ ALASKAN — ✚ PEGASUS — ❂ PERELANDRA

Pineapple Weed ✤ — freedom from injury/risk from calm awareness

Pink Monkeyflower ▲ — freedom to express true feelings after shame/fear

Purple Monkeyflower ▲ — creating own spiritual identity/values

Sagebrush ▲✚ — letting go, emptying and freeing oneself from excess attachment

Scarlet Monkeyflower ▲ — freedom to express powerful emotions openly/honestly

Sitka Burnet ✤ — freedom through healing the past on all levels

Spinach ■ — childlike joy, playfulness, freedom

Trumpet Vine ▲✚ — freedom to speak clearly/forcefully without holding back

Vetch ▼ — freedom from limitation

Walnut ●✚ — breaking free of limiting influences, especially from past circumstances

Wild Oat ● — overattachment to freedom, leading to lack of direction or purpose

Wild Potato Bush ◆ — freedom to move on in life

Frustration

Almond ■▲✚ — frustration, discontentment

Banksia Robur ◆ — frustration with life

Blackberry ■▲▼✚ — inability to manifest intentions into action

Blue Elf Viola ✤ — release of frustration

Daffodil ▲▼✚ — frustration of self-criticism

Gentian ●✚ — frustration from setback or failure

Green Rose ✚◗ — frustration, stagnation, repetition of mistakes

Impatiens ●✚ — frustration with the slowness of others

Indian Paintbrush ▲✚ — difficulty bringing vitality to creative expression

Iris ▲ — frustration in creative expression due to lack of inspiration

Penstemon ▲✚ — frustration with adversity, unexpected challenges

Rabbit Orchid ◗ — frustration with shallow, empty and obligatory relationships

Red Beak Orchid ◗ — adolescence/mid-life frustrations with duties and family ties

Silver Princess Gum, Gungurra ◗ — frustration when things don't work out

Snakebush ◗ — frustration from a lack of love
Wild Potato Bush ◆ — frustration with a sense of feeling weighed down
Ursinia ◗ — frustration with family or group
Ylang Ylang ✚ — calms anger, frustration, stress, depression
Yucca ✚ — transforms anger or frustration into spiritual energy
Zucchini ▲▼✚✺ — frustration, anger

Generosity

Blue Leschenaultia ◗ — rekindles the desire to give with grace and benevolence
Larkspur ▲✚ — leadership with cheerful/positive charisma, generosity, altruism
Peach ■▲✚ — self-involvement, thoughtlessness
Philotheca ◆ — excessive generosity, inability to accept acknowledgement
Raspberry ■✚ — kindness, compassion, empathy
Star Thistle ▲ — Generous, inclusive, giving/sharing, inner sense of abundance

Gentleness

Bachelor's Button ✚ — sense of gentleness/quiet with ability to express ideas
Banana ■▲▼✚ — calmness, stepping back and observing, non-reactiveness
Blackberry ■▲▼✚ — incisive, direct, yet gentle in speech
Calendula ▲▼✚ — caring, warmth, gentleness and receptivity
Deerbrush ▲ — gentle purity, clarity of purpose, sincerity of motivation
Dogwood ▲ — encourages gentleness, grace, and innocence in relationship
Flannel Flower ◆ — gentleness, sensitivity in touching, joy, trust, sensuality
Forget-Me-Not ▲✚✤ — being gentle with self
Northern Lady's Slipper ✤ — healing core traumas, touched by infinite gentleness
Pansy ▲✚ — maintaining gentleness, sense of beauty, possibility of renewal
Peach ■▲✚ — concern for welfare of others, empathy, nurturance

● BACH — ■ MASTER'S — ▲ FES — ▼ GREEN HOPE — ◆ AUSTRALIAN BUSH
◗ LIVING/AUSTRALIA — ✤ ALASKAN — ✚ PEGASUS — ✺ PERELANDRA

Plantain ▲ — to become gentler and more open to the ideas and wishes of others

Red Leschenaultia ❱ — essence of gentleness and sensitivity

Sitka Spruce Pollen ✤ — balancing power and gentleness in men and women

Sycamore ✚ — restores gentleness and smoothness to energy flow

Gloom

Baby Blue Eyes ▲▼ — gloom tinged with cynicism

Black Cohosh ▲ — profoundly dark states of mind, suspicion, brooding

Borage ▲▼✚ — uplifts the heart, dispels gloom and sorrow, gives courage

Cherry ■✚ — gloom, moodiness, grumpiness, ornery

Gorse ●✚ — despair, hopelessness about personal affairs

Mustard ●✚ — personal black cloud, sudden, unexpected feelings of gloom

Red Clover ▲▼ — easily influenced by projections of gloom/doom, group panic

Scotch Broom ▲✚ — depression about disasters/tragedies in the world

Gossip

Blackberry ■▲▼✚ — sarcasm, cynicism, tactlessness, gossiping

Fringed Mantis Orchid ❱ — can't resist gossiping

Grace

Angel's Trumpet ▲✚ — for soul to leave body peacefully and gracefully

Angelica ▲▼✚ — feeling in touch with the grace of the angelic realm

Blue Leschenaultia ❱ — rekindles the desire to give with grace and benevolence

Bougainvillaea ▼✚ — grace and beauty

Calendula ▲▼✚ — graceful receptivity to others

Deerbrush ▲ — purity of feelings within the heart

Dogwood ▲ — encourages gentleness, grace, and innocence in relationship

Holly ●✚ — extending grace and forgiveness to others

Jacaranda ◆ — softness and grace

Lotus ▲✚ — spiritual harmony, feeling of wholeness

● BACH — ■ MASTER'S — ▲ FES — ▼ GREEN HOPE — ◆ AUSTRALIAN BUSH
❱ LIVING/AUSTRALIA — ✤ ALASKAN — ✚ PEGASUS — ✪ PERELANDRA

Pine ● — ability to forgive oneself, to feel grace as a spiritual gift

Star Tulip ▲✚ — being in touch with the more feminine, graceful aspects of self

Thistle ▼ — to recognize grace in our lives

Vervain ●✚ — extreme intensity, fervency which robs one of grace and ease

Greed

Bluebell ◆ — fear of lack, greed

Chrysanthemum ▲✚ — monetary power as protection against mortality

Goldenrod ▲▼✚ — wanting material possessions to insure social status

Grape ■ — envy, greed, lust, jealousy

Peach ■▲✚ — selfishness, exploitativeness, "looking out for number one"

Sagebrush ▲✚ — overidentification with possessions/lifestyle

Star Thistle ▲ — lack of generosity, clinging to material possessions

Trillium ▲▼✚ — coveting the power/possessions of others, greed

Vine ●✚ — wanting leadership power for selfish ends

Grief

Artichoke ✚ — release grief and sadness

Bittersweet ✚ — releases grief, mourning and despondency

Bleeding Heart ▲✚ — to release an ended relationship or death of a loved one

Borage ▲▼✚ — uplifts the heart, dispels gloom and sorrow, gives courage

Cape Honeysuckle ✚ — balancing grief, loneliness, or other difficult emotion states

Dampiera ◗ — letting go and letting life flow

Dandelion ▲▼✚❖ — release of emotional/grief blockages stuck in body

Dill ▲▼❂ — grief with denial of self, of feelings

Eucalyptus ▲✚ — eases grief, hostilities, and difficulties in partnerships

Evening Primrose ▲ — deep soul pain, traumatic abuse in early childhood

Fennel ✚ — indecisive, depressed and subject to grief

Forget-Me-Not ▲✚❖ — to remember friends who have passed away

Golden Ear Drops ▲ — releasing tears of grief held back since childhood

Hawthorne ✚ — brings hope, protecting spirit in stress, pain or grief
Honeysuckle ●✚ — letting go of the past
Hyssop ▲▼✚ — grief with feelings of guilt
Judas Tree ✚ — gets one beyond grief, remorse and depression
Love-Lies-Bleeding ▲ — profound melancholia and anguish, especially private suffering
Milk Thistle ✚ — grief and hysteria
Mulberry-Red ✚ — alleviates grief, mourning, may restimulate sense of purpose
Pansy ▲✚ — grief over past loves, loss of a loved one
Pear ■▲▼✚ — extreme grief
Pleurisy Root ✚ — suppressed rage and grief
Radish ▼✚ — bereavement with an inability to cope
Sagebrush ▲✚ — accepting the pain and emptiness of any kind of loss
Star of Bethlehem ●▼◗ — soothing/calming after shock of death or tragedy
Sturt Desert Pea ◆ — deep hurt, sadness, emotional pain
Wild Rose ● — withdrawal/numbing due to grief
Yerba Santa ▲✚ — deep melancholia, feelings of wasting away, deterioration

Groundedness

Alpine Lily ▲ — disconnected from female body
Buttercup ▲✚ — well grounded and appreciative of life's riches and pleasures
California Wild Rose ▲✚ — difficulty coming into the body
Canyon Dudleya ▲ — difficulty accepting ordinary/mundane reality
Clematis ●✚ — being present in the here and now, those who feel "floaty"
Cow Parsnip ❖ — connecting to place
Corn ■▲▼✚✪ — bringing spirituality through the body and into the earth
Eucalyptus ▲✚ — eases grief, hostilities, and difficulties in partnerships
Fawn Lily ▲ — bring spiritual forces into earthly life, especially with tendency to retreat
Fireweed ▲❖✚ — grounding, cleansing old energy patterns
Golden Yarrow ▲ — staying embodied

Hibiscus ▲ — experiencing sexuality as a positive expression of the body

Indian Paintbrush ▲✚ — igniting forces of vitality for higher/creative work

Lady's Slipper ▲✣ — spiritual forces not fully grounded and integrated

Manzanita ▲✚ — feeling at home in the physical body and earthly world

Queen Anne's Lace ▲▼✚ — distorted psychic forces from unstable feelings

Red Lily ◆ — grounded, focused, living in the present

Rosemary ▲▼✚ — tendency to overly discarnate states

St. John's Wort ▲▼✚ — protection when consciousness too open/expanded

Shooting Star ▲✚✣ — feeling at home, overcoming deep-seated alienation

Strawberry ■▲✚ — being ungrounded

Sundew ◆ — daydreaming, procrastinating, disconnected, spaced out, lack of focus

Sweet Pea ▲✚ — finding roots in community life, developing sense of place

Vervain ●✚ — zealous/fanatic activity which overrides body awareness

Group Dynamics (see Community Life)

Guilt

Bo Tree ✚ — guilt from lack of spiritual path

Deerbrush ▲ — mixed motives, unclear intentions

Elm ●✚ — guilt/misery when can't measure up to expectations

Eucalyptus ▲✚ — eases grief, guilt, and difficulties in partnerships

Golden Ear Drops ▲ — repressed guilt from childhood

Mullein ▲✚ — listening to the voice of conscience

Peach ■▲✚ — guilt with an inability to receive love

Pine ● — self-blame

Pink Monkeyflower ▲ — covering up, fear of exposure, profound shame

Pink Yarrow ▲ — undue guilt, emerging merging with others resulting in guilt

Strawberry ■▲✚ — guilt stemming from a dysfunctional childhood

Sturt Desert Rose ◆ — guilt, feeling bad about self from previous action

Habit Patterns

Almond ■▲✚ — making wrong choices from the power of past habits

Blue China Orchid ◗ — breaking the spell of habitual patterns of behavior

Cayenne ▲✚ — breaking free of habitual behavior, fiery catalyst for change

Chestnut Bud ●✚ — constant repetition of experiences without learning from them

Crab Apple ●▼✚ — to break bad habits

Morning Glory ▲▼✚ — to overcome destructive habits

Rice ✚ — habits related to discipline needs like smoking, sadomasochism

Rock Water ● — overly strict, unyielding habits from extreme ideals/discipline

Sagebrush ▲✚ — breaking free of old identities and habits

Walnut ●✚ — letting go of habits/lifestyle patterns taken from influence of others

White Nicotiana ▼ — cleansing ego habits and cravings

Hallucinations

Amaranthus ✚ — calms disruptive dream states, hallucinations

Lima Bean ✚ — eases hallucinations

Happiness

Apple ■▲✚ — hope, motivation, a positive outlook

Borage ▲▼✚ — uplifts the heart, dispels gloom and sorrow, gives courage

Cherry ■✚ — inspiration to others, optimistic, positive

Fringed Lily Twiner ◗ — love/focus toward others, one becomes happy by giving

Mountain Devil ◆ — unconditional love, forgiveness, happiness, inner peace

Rosemary ▲▼✚ — happiness, sensitivity and sentiment

Star of Bethlehem ●▼◗ — a sense of inner divinity

Sunshine Wattle ◆ — acceptance of the beauty and joy in the present, optimism

Tuberose ✚ — opens the heart to receive love and happiness

● BACH — ■ MASTER'S — ▲ FES — ▼ GREEN HOPE — ◆ AUSTRALIAN BUSH
◗ LIVING/AUSTRALIA — ❖ ALASKAN — ✚ PEGASUS — ✪ PERELANDRA

Valerian ▲✚ — to bring tranquility and peace

Vanda Orchid ▼ — to bring hope and happiness

Hardness

Baby Blue Eyes ▲▼ — hard, numb exterior, cynical, bitter attitude

Beech ●✚ — hard, judgemental, demanding, unrealistic perfectionism

Dandelion ▲▼✚❖ — extreme tension from overactivity leading to hardness

Dogwood ▲ — hard, limiting emotions, self-abusive, accident-prone/self-destructive

Giant Redwood ▼ — too hard on self

Morning Glory ▲▼✚ — harsh lifestyle, habits which are hard on body

Nicotiana ▲ — appearance of hard exterior/tough posture, macho

Oak ●✚ — strong, unyielding, not knowing when to surrender

Orange Leschenaultia ◗ — gradually closing up/desensitizing from harsh realities

Pine ● — hard attitude toward self, extreme self-judgement/blame

Pink Monkeyflower ▲ — inability to be vulnerable due to shame, rejection

Pixie Mops ◗ — hardened after being let down

Poison Oak ▲ — creating a hard exterior, can't show vulnerability, hostility

Quince ▲✚ — integrating the softer, feminine aspect when also needing to be strong

Red Leschenaultia ◗ — discourages harshness or hard-heartedness

Rock Water ● — overly strict, unyielding habits from extreme ideals/discipline

Star Tulip ▲✚ — softening of soul forces

Harmony

Angelica ▲▼✚ — feeling in touch with the grace of the angelic realm

California Poppy ▲▼ — feeling harmony within self

Chamomile ▲✚ — to restore emotional harmony after upset

Corn ■▲▼✚✪ — harmony in diversity

Fuchsia ▲ — bring repressed emotions to awareness to be harmonized

Fun Orchid ✚ — dancing, laughing, harmony, love, angels

Jacob's Ladder ❖✚ — familial harmony

Lavender ▲✚ — emotional calming

● BACH — ■ MASTER'S — ▲ FES — ▼ GREEN HOPE — ◆ AUSTRALIAN BUSH
◗ LIVING/AUSTRALIA — ❖ ALASKAN — ✚ PEGASUS — ✪ PERELANDRA

Lotus ▲✚ — spiritual harmony, feeling of wholeness

Pear ■▲▼✚ — returns a sense of rhythm and proportion

Pineapple Weed ❖ — harmony between mothers and children

Quaking Grass ▲✚ — creating harmony within a group

Shasta Daisy ▲ — creating harmonious patterns in work and thinking

Soapberry ❖ — balancing one's personal power with the power of nature

Spruce ▲✚ — harmony to those not accepting questioning themselves

Star Tulip ▲✚ — harmony in relationship of soul to spiritual world

Sweet Pea ▲✚ — social harmony

Venus Orchid ✚ — harmony, tenderness, understanding the Yin of our being

Watermelon ▲✚ — harmony between a couple desiring to have a child

Hate

Black Cohosh ▲ — twisted love or love-hate relationships, tending toward violence

Black Kangaroo Paw ◗ — grief/anger obsessive cycles

Cape Bluebell ◗ — for issues of the past that leave a bitter taste

Coriander ✚ — hatred transformed into passion

Crab Apple ●▼✚ — self-hate, especially with obsession over impurity/contamination

Holly ●✚ — hostility toward others out of jealousy, sibling rivalry, etc

Mountain Devil ◆ — hatred, jealousy, holding grudges, suspicion

Oregon Grape ▲ — expecting hate from others

Pine ● — undue blame and hatred of oneself, unable to accept own mistakes

Scarlet Monkeyflower ▲ — explosive emotions from powerlessness, suppressed rage

Snapdragon ▲▼✚ — verbal criticism/abuse, misplaced aggression

Willow ●✚ — resentment, blame of others, hatred over time turning to bitterness

Haughtiness (see Aloofness)

Healers

Agrimony ●✚ — attachment to image of healer as one who is beyond pain

● BACH — ■ MASTER'S — ▲ FES — ▼ GREEN HOPE — ◆ AUSTRALIAN BUSH
◗ LIVING/AUSTRALIA — ❖ ALASKAN — ✚ PEGASUS — ✪ PERELANDRA

Calendula ▲▼✚ — graceful receptivity to others, ability to listen

Calla Lily ▲✚ — enhances compassion for self

Carob (St. John's Bread) ✚ — empathy, group interaction

Centaury ● — drained/depleted rather than replenished by healing work

Deerbrush ▲ — recognizing/applying true higher motives for healing work

Eyebright ✚ — for psychic healer/practitioner to better perceive condition of client

Golden Yarrow ▲ — receptive/engaged in healing process without vulnerability

Impatiens ●✚ — inability to be receptive to client's true needs, overscheduling

Lime ▼✚ — to improve healer's ability to heal

Mahogany ✚ — grounding, release negative thoughts

Mallow ▲▼✚ — conveying qualities of personal warmth/nurturing in healing

Maple (Sugar) ✚ — empathy between healer and client improves, aids acupuncturists

Mariposa Lily ▲ — imparting feminine forces of nurturing and care

Oak ●✚ — taking on role of healer as hero, needing to learn to set limits

Pink Monkeyflower ▲ — fear of self-exposure or vulnerability

Pink Yarrow ▲ — tendency toward emotional merging with others

Quinoa ✚ — grounding, gets people beyond power trips

Red Chestnut ●✚ — excessive worry/anxiety about well-being of clients

Rosa Hemisphaerica ✚ — increases healers ability to generate energy

Rosa Xanthina ✚ — helps healers remove negativity

Self-Heal ▲ — contacting true inner healing capabilities

Shasta Daisy ▲ — ability to think holistically about client's condition

Skullcap ✚ — empathy and compassion in the healing process

Snowplant ✚ — deeper understanding of incoming light and energy

Sunflower ▲▼✚✤ — conveying warm radiance from within

Witch Hazel ▲✚ — for energy healers

Yarrow ▲ — overabsorption of others' suffering, feeling depleted

Yellow Star Tulip ▲ — compassionate presence

Zinnia ▲▼✚✪ — bringing humor/light-heartedness to healing approach

---

● BACH — ■ MASTER'S — ▲ FES — ▼ GREEN HOPE — ◆ AUSTRALIAN BUSH
◗ LIVING/AUSTRALIA — ✤ ALASKAN — ✚ PEGASUS — ✪ PERELANDRA

Healing Process

Agrimony ●✚ — denial of pain or of the need for healing

Angelica ▲▼✚ — protection/nurturing from spiritual guides

Arnica ▲✚ — releasing armoring from parts deeply wounded/traumatized

Black-Eyed Susan ▲▼♦ — for any form of denial during healing process

Borage ▲▼✚ — uplifts the heart, dispels gloom and sorrow, gives courage

California Wild Rose ▲✚ — inability to be full committed to healing, apathy

Canyon Dudleya ▲ — overdramatizing healing or suffering

Cerato ●✚ — following own guidance in healing process

Chestnut Bud ●✚ — to break repeated pattern in illness

Crab Apple ●▼✚ — when obsessed with healing, especially need for cleansing/purification

Echinacea ▲✚ — re-building core self after trauma, surgery, devastation

Fairy Lantern ▲ — regressive tendencies in therapeutic process

Fuchsia ▲ — psychosomatic symptoms masking real pain and suffering

Gentian ●✚ — frustration from setback or failure

Golden Ear Drops ▲ — contacting painful memories

Gorse ●✚ — attachment to suffering, extreme melancholy or depression

Heather ●✚ — obsession with one's symptoms, compulsion to talk about problems

Impatiens ●✚ — unwilling to accept slow process of healing journey

Lavender ▲✚ — emotional calming

Love-Lies-Bleeding ▲ — finding meaning in one's suffering

Manzanita ▲✚ — difficulty integrating bodily component into healing work

Mariposa Lily ▲ — contacting core feelings from childhood

Milkweed ▲✚ — extreme dependency

Mountain Pennyroyal ▲ — cleansing toxic thoughts

Mustard ●✚ — accepting the dark as well as the light

Olive ●✚ — depletion of vitality after long illness/struggle

Penstemon ▲✚ — frustration with adversity, unexpected challenges

Pine ● — hard attitude toward self, extreme self-judgement/blame

● BACH — ■ MASTER'S — ▲ FES — ▼ GREEN HOPE — ♦ AUSTRALIAN BUSH
❿ LIVING/AUSTRALIA — ❖ ALASKAN — ✚ PEGASUS — ✪ PERELANDRA

Pink Monkeyflower ▲ — difficulty letting down barriers or letting others help

Pink Yarrow ▲ — hypersensitive to the healing process

Pretty Face ▲ — willingness to go through period of ugliness/discomfort

Rosemary ▲▼✚ — unable to be present in physical body

Sagebrush ▲✚ — willingness to go through stage of aloneness/emptiness

Self-Heal ▲ — contacting true inner healing capabilities

Shasta Daisy ▲ — to integrate different therapeutic approaches

Sunflower ▲▼✚❖ — balancing ego forces between self-image/self-examination

Walnut ●✚ — making major transitions in the healing process

Wild Rose ● — apathy/resignation when faced with illness/challenge

Yerba Santa ▲✚ — releasing emotional congestion in the heart

Heart

Aloe Vera ▲▼✚ — replenishing creative forces of the heart

Alpine Azalea ❖ — opening heart to loving energy of the planet

Alpine Lily ▲ — for women: integrating heart feelings with female organ feelings

Baby Blue Eyes ▲▼ — opening heart to loving presence of spiritual world

Bleeding Heart ▲✚ — to release an ended relationship or death of a loved one

Bluebell ◆ — opens the heart, joy, sharing

Borage ▲▼✚ — uplifts the heart, dispels gloom and sorrow, gives courage

California Wild Rose ▲✚ — strengthening/vitalizing the heart

Carnation ✚ — purity and love

Cherry ■✚ — inspiration to others, optimistic, positive

Dandelion ▲▼✚❖ — overachiever, bringing balance to the heart

Fawn Lily ▲ — bring spiritual forces into earthly life, especially with tendency to retreat

Forget-Me-Not ▲✚❖ — spiritualizing the love currents of the heart

Foxglove ▲❖✚ — to see through perceptual constrictions to the 'heart' of the matter

Grape ■ — loving without condition, demand or expectation

Green Bog Orchid ❖ — release of pain and fear held deep in the heart

Green Fairy Orchid ❖ — balancing male and female energies in the heart

Harebell ❖ — bringing unconditional love through the heart

Hawthorne ✚ — cleanses the heart of negativity

Heart Orchid ✚ — heart energy, love, endless love

Holly ●✚ — hostility toward others out of jealousy, sibling rivalry, etc

Hollyhock ▲✚ — open, compassionate heart

Impatiens ●✚ — frenetic, over-impulsive, fast-pace causing stress on heart

Lamb's Quarters ❖ — balance between the heart and mind

Love-Lies-Bleeding ▲ — finding meaning in one's suffering

Love Orchid ✚ — heart opening, love energy, healing

Mariposa Lily ▲ — receptive to human love, maternal nurturing, ability to mother

Nicotiana ▲ — to counteract stimulants or other physical measures to rouse heart

Pink Powder Puff ✚ — heart awakening

Peony ▲✚ — forgiveness and compassion

Pink Everlasting ◗ — restoring milk of human kindness to hearts

Pink Monkeyflower ▲ — allowing feelings to flow through heart more easily

Pink Yarrow ▲ — to distinguish compassion from overly sympathetic merging

Pixie Mops ◗ — strengthens heart so one does not become like those resented

Raspberry ■✚ — kindness, compassion, empathy

Red Leschenaultia ◗ — discourages harshness or hard-heartedness

Tree Peony ▼ — unconditional and total love

Tundra Twayblade ❖ — completely releasing impact of abuse

Yellow Star Tulip ▲ — following your heart

Yerba Santa ▲✚ — releasing emotional congestion in the heart

Hesitation

Cerato ●✚ — uncertainty about values, over-dependent on advice

Fairy Lantern ▲ — waiting for others to take responsibility, helplessness

Larch ●✚ — uncertainty, lack of confidence

Menzies Banksia ◗ — hesitation from fear of being emotionally hurt

Mimulus ●✚ — holding back due to fears of everyday life

Queensland Bottlebrush ◗ — healthy flow of energy, enjoy people without hesitation

Scleranthus ●✚ — fluctuating between two possibilities when making decisions

Tansy ▲✚ — difficulty being decisive, lethargic

Tomato ■▼✚✪ — minor hesitation to severe terror

Home and Lifestyle

Beech ●✚ — hypersensitivity in home, compulsion for order, intolerance

Buttercup ▲✚ — feeling worthless or low self-esteem in domestic role

Canyon Dudleya ▲ — inability to identify with ordinary household tasks

Crab Apple ●▼✚ — compulsive cleaning and putting things in order

Fairy Lantern ▲ — inability to face world/work: living at home for too long

Fawn Lily ▲ — treating home as a retreat

Filaree ▲✚ — attachment to mundane aspects of household, such as cleaning

Honeysuckle ●✚ — home filled with nostalgia/memorabilia to an extreme

Impatiens ●✚ — performing household tasks quickly, irritably

Indian Pink ▲✚ — scattered/disheveled environment, quick pace

Iris ▲ — dull, drab or ugly living environment, excessive use of TV

Madia ▲✚ — inability to complete simple tasks, easily distracted

Mariposa Lily ▲ — to bring maternal warmth and nurturing presence

Mimulus ●✚ — being housebound or shut in

Morning Glory ▲▼✚ — chaotic lifestyle or living environment due to erratic habits

Mountain Pennyroyal ▲ — to purify home or environment from disturbed thoughts

Pink Yarrow ▲ — oversensitivity/emotional merging with environment

Pretty Face ▲ — desire for home to appear beautiful in conformance to others

Sagebrush ▲✚ — purifying and simplifying lifestyle

● BACH — ■ MASTER'S — ▲ FES — ▼ GREEN HOPE — ◆ AUSTRALIAN BUSH
◗ LIVING/AUSTRALIA — ❖ ALASKAN — ✚ PEGASUS — ✪ PERELANDRA

Shasta Daisy ▲ — bringing harmony to chaotic home
Star Tulip ▲✚ — developing quiet inner presence in home
Sweet Pea ▲✚ — homelessness of social isolation, moving frequently
Tansy ▲✚ — inability to complete household tasks, lethargy, procrastination
Walnut ●✚ — moving, changing living situation
Yucca ✚ — fear of leaving home town
Zinnia ▲▼✚⊙ — finding joy/interest even in mundane tasks

Honesty

Agrimony ●✚ — acknowledging inner conflict, covering up true feelings
Black-Eyed Susan ▲▼◆ — to counteract denial
Blackberry ■▲▼✚ — purity of thought
California Poppy ▲▼ — looking honestly within oneself instead of escapism
Calypso Orchid ✚ — wonderment, honesty, availability, openness, commonality
Canyon Dudleya ▲ — inflation of psychic experiences, compulsion to exaggerate
Coconut ■ — honesty without excuses
Fuchsia ▲ — expressing basic emotions rather than false emotionality
Goldenrod ▲▼✚ — conforming to win approval
Mullein ▲✚ — listening to the voice of conscience
Pink Monkeyflower ▲ — showing true feeling despite fear
Pineapple ■✚ — honesty with self-assuredness
Sagebrush ▲✚ — inappropriate identity or self-image which needs to be released
Scarlet Monkeyflower ▲ — recognition/proper expression of powerful emotions
Snapdragon ▲▼✚ — contacting core feelings of anger/sexuality when aggressive
Spiderwort ✚ — honesty and clarity
Spinach ■ — honesty with childlike joy

Hope

Apple ■▲✚ — hope, motivation, a positive outlook
Beech ●✚ — seeing the good in each person and situation

Birch ▲✚ — hope for the future
Blackthorn ▲ — hope and joy
Cherry ■✚ — inspiration to others, optimistic, positive
Gorse ●✚ — deep abiding faith and hope
Orange ■ — energy, renewed interest in life
Star of Bethlehem ●▼◗ — a sense of inner divinity
Sunshine Wattle ◆ — acceptance of the beauty and joy in the present, optimism
Sweet Chestnut ●✚ — restoring faith when stretched beyond limits
Tomato ■▼✚✪ — knowing there is no failure
Waratah ◆ — courage, tenacity, faith, adaptability, survival skills

Hostility

Baby Blue Eyes ▲▼ — detached hostility masking as cynicism
Beech ●✚ — hostility expressed as criticism or condemnation of others
Holly ●✚ — hostility toward others out of jealousy, rivalry, etc
Oregon Grape ▲ — expecting hostility from others, paranoia
Poison Oak ▲ — creating a hard exterior, can't show vulnerability, hostility
Snapdragon ▲▼✚ — verbal criticism/abuse, misplaced aggression
Tiger Lily ▲✚ — transmuting hostile or aggressive tendencies

Humor

Bird of Paradise ✚ — freedom, establishing a sense of humor
Blackberry ■▲▼✚ — sarcasm, cynicism, tactlessness, gossiping
Fig ■▲✚ — sense of humor, ability to "go with the flow"
Larkspur ▲✚ — humorous, cooperative, caring, playful, friendly, mellow
Little Flannel Flower ◆ — playfulness, joyful, ability to have fun, spontaneity
Spinach ■ — childlike joy, playfulness, freedom
Valerian ▲✚ — promotes relaxation, contentment
Zinnia ▲▼✚✪ — to encourage exuberance, joyful involvement in life

Hurt

Aloe Vera ▲▼✚ — replenishing creative forces of the heart
California Wild Rose ▲✚ — acceptance of painful feelings in the heart

Catspaw ❱ — to express hurt feelings, bringing reality to obligatory relationships

Chamomile ▲✚ — to restore emotional harmony after upset

Comfrey ▲▼✚✪ — supports healing on all levels

Cotton Grass ✤ — letting go of pain held in the body

Golden Ear Drops ▲ — contacting painful memories

Illyarrie ❱ — to deal with past shadows and pain

Ladies' Tresses ✤ — for releasing deeply held traumas

Mauve Melaleuca ❱ — despondent from sadness and great hurt

Menzies Banksia ❱ — fear of being emotionally hurt

Pink Monkeyflower ▲ — freedom to express true feelings after shame/fear

Pink Mulla Mulla ◆ — deep hurt

Raspberry ■✚ — "turning the other cheek," releasing old wounds, forgiveness

River Beauty ✤ — emotional re-orientation and recovery after shock

Sturt Desert Pea ◆ — deep hurt, sadness, emotional pain

Valerian ▲✚ — promotes relaxation, contentment

Violet Butterfly ❱ — emotionally shattered during/after relationship traumas

White Fireweed ✤ — recovery from emergency

Yerba Santa ▲✚ — releasing emotional congestion in the heart

Hyperactivity

Black-Eyed Susan ▲▼◆ — rushing, always on the go, impatient, lack of inner peace

Chamomile ▲✚ — emotional hyperactivity

Cherry Plum ●✚ — out of control, erratic or destructive behavior

Impatiens ●✚ — difficulty paying attention, restlessness, unable to focus

Jacaranda ◆ — scattered, changeable, dithering, unfocused, rushing

Licorice ✚ — calms restlessness

Loofa (Lufa) ▲✚ — hyperactivity, defines skin as the space of the physical body

Madia ▲✚ — short attention span, flits from one activity to another

Morning Glory ▲▼✚ — erratic eating, sleeping rhythms, difficulty rising

Petunia ▲✚ — hyperactivity, stuttering, forgetfulness

Vervain ●✚ — zealous/fanatic activity, abundance of energy

Hypochondria

Apple ■▲✛ — fear of illness, hypochondria

Elecampagne ✛ — hypochondria and stress

Fig ■▲✛ — fanaticism, too strict a discipline

Fuchsia ▲ — psychosomatic symptoms masking real pain and suffering

Heather ●✛ — obsession with one's symptoms, compulsion to talk about problems

Peach Flowered Tea Tree ◆ — hypochondria, taking responsibility for own health

Hysteria

Basil ▲✛✪ — eases anxiety by getting to the core of the cause of hysteria

Canyon Dudleya ▲ — exaggerated emotions

Chamomile ▲✛ — extreme emotional upset

Cherry Plum ●✛ — out of control, erratic or destructive behavior

Cosmos ▲▼✛ — overexcited mental activity, rapid, inarticulate speech

Fuchsia ▲ — false emotionality

Milk Thistle ✛ — grief and hysteria

Mugwort ▲✛ — overemphasis on psychic life which leads to emotional imbalance

Pink Yarrow ▲ — pathological merging with others' emotions

Purple Monkeyflower ▲ — profound fear or panic

Red Clover ▲▼ — easily influenced by projections of gloom/doom, group panic

Rescue Remedy (Five Flower Formula) ● — to bring immediate calming

Rock Rose ●✛ — panic/hysteria in extreme situations, facing death/destruction

Rose-Honorine de Brabant ✛ — elimination of stress, hysteria, anxiety

Ideals

Beech ●✛ — overly perfectionist ideals, harsh standards imposed on others

Blackberry ■▲▼✛ — bringing ideals into practical manifestation

California Wild Rose ▲✛ — activation of true ideals

Centaury ● — wanting to be of service, inner balance between own/others' needs

---

● BACH — ■ MASTER'S — ▲ FES — ▼ GREEN HOPE — ◆ AUSTRALIAN BUSH
❧ LIVING/AUSTRALIA — ✤ ALASKAN — ✛ PEGASUS — ✪ PERELANDRA

Clematis ●✚ — impractical ideals and visions, dreaminess

Fawn Lily ▲ — strong spiritual ideals that need to be shared with others

Larkspur ▲✚ — positive idealism, altruistic leadership

Mauve Melaleuca ◗ — the realization that idealism about love is important

Mountain Pride ▲✚ — ability to speak out for one's ideals, active commitment

Periwinkle ✚ — integrates personal philosophy/ideals with higher spiritual concepts

Pink Impatiens ◗ — strength of convictions, creative will

Rock Water ● — overly strict ideals for oneself and others, inflexible idealism

Ursinia ◗ — to retain idealism

Vervain ●✚ — strongly held ideals/beliefs which can lead to fanaticism

Wooly Banksia ◗ — desire to pursue ideals/goals when struggle seems too much

Identity Crisis

Black Currant ▼ — deep fears related to identity shifts and crises

Columbine ✤ — building a strong projection of one's identity

Milkweed ▲✚ — coping independently and without escaping

Monkshood ▲✚✤ — lack of boundaries from a weak spiritual identity

Papaya ▲▼✚ — helps resolve identity crises connected with one's sexuality

Pineapple ■✚ — contentment with self

Tamarack ✤ — awareness of true essence, self-confidence/ understanding abilities

Quaking Grass ▲✚ — to balance individuality with its social identity

Yellow Dryas ✤ — confidence from knowing one's greater identity

Immaturity

Fairy Lantern ▲ — fear of growing up, of adult identity

Indian Paintbrush ▲✚ — emotional immaturity

Plantain ▲ — immaturity, afraid to grow up, apprehension

● BACH — ■ MASTER'S — ▲ FES — ▼ GREEN HOPE — ◆ AUSTRALIAN BUSH
◗ LIVING/AUSTRALIA — ✤ ALASKAN — ✚ PEGASUS — ✪ PERELANDRA

Immobility

Blackberry ■▲▼✚ — unproductive thought patterns

Cayenne ▲✚ — fiery catalyst for change

Golden Yarrow ▲ — performance anxiety, wanting to act but too sensitive

Iris ▲ — lack of inspiration

Larch ●✚ — paralysis due to fear of failure, inability to take risks

Morning Glory ▲▼✚ — erratic habits, addictions

Rock Rose ●✚ — paralyzed by fear of death or destruction

Scleranthus ●✚ — inability to make a decision, thus preventing forward movement

Tansy ▲✚ — sluggish, lethargic, overly phlegmatic, indecisive

Thistle ▼ — immobility, powerlessness, flight/fright syndrome

Wild Oat ● — avoiding commitment to life purpose/work goals

Impatience

Black-Eyed Susan ▲▼◆ — rushing, always on the go, impatient, lack of inner peace

Calendula ▲▼✚ — difficulty listening

Cosmos ▲▼✚ — to regulate the flow of thoughts, too rapid speech/thinking patterns

Impatiens ●✚ — expecting others to go faster, impatience

Cow Parsnip ✤ — eases impatience, dissatisfaction and anxiety during life changes

Poison Oak ▲ — susceptible to irritation/anger, antipathetic versus sympathetic

Impetuousness

Impatiens ●✚ — frenetic, over-impulsive

Kangaroo Paw ◆ — unaware of appropriate social behavior

Inadequacy

Buttercup ▲✚ — feeling vocation/contribution does not count

Elm ●✚ — feeling inadequate to one's responsibilities

Evening Primrose ▲ — feeling unlovable/unwanted from childhood rejection/abuse

Fairy Lantern ▲ — feeling one cannot cope with adult responsibilities

---

● BACH — ■ MASTER'S — ▲ FES — ▼ GREEN HOPE — ◆ AUSTRALIAN BUSH
❱ LIVING/AUSTRALIA — ✤ ALASKAN — ✚ PEGASUS — ✪ PERELANDRA

Golden Yarrow ▲ — performance anxiety, overanxious, oversensitive

Goldenrod ▲▼✚ — socially insecure, trying to measure up to others' standards

Iris ▲ — feeling uncreative

Larch ●✚ — self-censorship, fear of failure, of being judged as inadequate

Milkweed ▲✚ — unable to cope with life or normal ego demands, dependency

Peach ■▲✚ — inability to relate to others' realities

Peony ▲✚ — dispels feelings of inadequacy

Pine ● — hard attitude toward self, extreme self-judgement/blame

Pink Monkeyflower ▲ — sense of shame

Pretty Face ▲ — never feeling beautiful enough

Star Thistle ▲ — fear of lack

Sticky Monkeyflower ▲ — feelings of sexual inadequacy/awkwardness

Strawberry ■▲✚ — need for approval

Sunflower ▲▼✚❖ — self-effacement, lack of balanced ego forces

Indecision

Apple ■▲✚ — to integrate desires and willpower to realize goals and visions

Blackberry ■▲▼✚ — inability to manifest intentions into action

Cayenne ▲✚ — cutting through stagnation or indecision

Cerato ●✚ — inability to make decisions, overly reliant on advice of others

Coffee ▲✚ — helps overly analytical people make quick decisions

Fennel ✚ — indecisive, depressed and subject to grief

Jacaranda ◆ — scattered, changeable, dithering, unfocused, rushing

Larch ●✚ — uncertainty, lack of confidence

Lettuce ■✚ — indecisive, emotional congestion

Mullein ▲✚ — inability to connect with inner guidance/find inner values

Nutmeg ✚ — uncertainty, attunement to higher self

Paw Paw ✚◆ — lack of focus and clarity

Red Lily ◆ — vagueness, indecisiveness, daydreaming

Scleranthus ●✚ — fluctuating between two possibilities when making decisions

Sticky Geranium ❖ — focused and decisive action

Strawberry ■▲✚ — need for approval

Sundew ◆ — daydreaming, procrastinating, disconnected, spaced out, lack of focus

Tansy ▲✚ — procrastinating, lethargic, overly phlegmatic, indecisive

Wild Oat ● — avoiding commitment to life purpose/work goals

Independence

Angelsword ◆ — spiritual discernment

Bleeding Heart ▲✚ — emotional freedom, ending co-dependent tendencies

Evening Primrose ▲ — feeling unsafe so unable to be independent

Fairy Lantern ▲ — healthy maturation, acceptance of adult responsibilities

Milkweed ▲✚ — coping independently and without escaping

Southern Cross ◆❱ — personal power, positive attitude, taking responsibility

Individuality

Bougainvillaea ▼✚ — promotes free expression of individuality

Centaury ● — suppression of true individuality to serve the needs of others

Chrysanthemum ▲✚ — contacting one's true spiritual self

Echinacea ▲✚ — reclaiming one's integrity/dignity despite prior abuse/trauma

Fairy Lantern ▲ — cultivating more individuality by taking adult responsibility

Goldenrod ▲▼✚ — balance between group identity and individual identity

Milkweed ▲✚ — poorly integrated individuality, blotting out/obliterating ego

Mullein ▲✚ — fulfillment of true potential

Purple Monkeyflower ▲ — developing spiritual identity, after stifling from fear

Sagebrush ▲✚ — ability to reflect about and observe the self

Self-Heal ▲ — contacting inner resources, self-reliance

Sunflower ▲▼✚❖ — general remedy to stimulate positive individuality

---

● BACH — ■ MASTER'S — ▲ FES — ▼ GREEN HOPE — ◆ AUSTRALIAN BUSH
❱ LIVING/AUSTRALIA — ❖ ALASKAN — ✚ PEGASUS — ✪ PERELANDRA

Violet ▲ — fear of losing individuality in group, tendency to shyness/retreat

Inertia

Baby Blue Eyes ▲▼ — cynicism numbing the soul's awareness

Blackberry ■▲▼✛ — inability to manifest intentions into action

Cayenne ▲✛ — cutting through stagnation or indecision

Chestnut Bud ●✛ — not learning from life lessons

Morning Glory ▲▼✛ — getting stuck in destructive, addictive habit patterns

Tansy ▲✛ — procrastinating, lethargic, overly phlegmatic, indecisive

White Chestnut ● — stuck in a mental rut, "broken record" of repeating thoughts

Inferiority

Basil ▲✛✪ — inferiority complex

Buttercup ▲✛ — feeling vocation/contribution does not count

Cowslip Orchid ❱ — feeling inferior from other's success

Hibbertia ◆ — rigid personality, fanaticism about self-improvement

Pineapple ■✛ — contentment with self

Urchin Dryandra ❱ — self worth, understanding of how one got into victimhood

Watermelon ▲✛ — easing of obsessive and depressed states

Yellow Cone Flower ❱ — most important opinion is the one of yourself

Influence

Angelica ▲▼✛ — ability to receive positive influence/guidance from spiritual world

Centaury ● — excessively influenced by others

Cerato ●✛ — inability to make decisions, overly reliant on advice of others

Garlic ▲✛ — increased susceptibility to parasitic influence, weakened by fear/anxiety

Larkspur ▲✛ — influencing others through balanced leadership, positive charisma

Mountain Pride ▲✛ — clearing mind of negative thoughts taken on from others

Pink Yarrow ▲ — absorbing or acting out thoughts/feelings of others

---

● BACH — ■ MASTER'S — ▲ FES — ▼ GREEN HOPE — ◆ AUSTRALIAN BUSH
❱ LIVING/AUSTRALIA — ✤ ALASKAN — ✛ PEGASUS — ✪ PERELANDRA

Vervain ●✚ — intense and overbearing influence on others
Vine ●✚ — influencing others adversely, strong willed
Walnut ●✚ — breaking free from cultural/family influences

Inherited Behavior

Agave Yaquinana ✚ — beliefs about separation, loneliness, etc. from past-lives
Black Cohosh ▲ — abusive, exploitative, incestuous relationships
Boab ◆ — release of abusive thought patterns from family
Fireweed ▲❖✚ — cleansing old energy patterns
Larch ●✚ — clears old patterns of limitation

Inhibition

Catnip ✚ — social inhibitions
Fig ■▲✚ — rigidity, self-limitation, too strict a discipline
Penstemon ▲✚ — sexual shyness and inhibition
Tomato ■▼✚✪ — fear, withdrawal, shyness

Initiative

Blackberry ■▲▼✚ — putting ideas into action, overcoming inertia
Corn ■▲▼✚✪ — taking initiative in projects

Inner Child

Alpine Lily ▲ — rejection of/alienation from feminine/mother or mother role
Angelica ▲▼✚ — ability to receive positive influence/guidance from spiritual world
Baby Blue Eyes ▲▼ — mistrust from abandonment/estrangement from father
Balsam Poplar ❖ — healing sexual issues
Beech ●✚ — critical judgement of others, judgement of the childlike aspects of self
Black-Eyed Susan ▲▼◆ — recalling buried painful experiences from childhood
Bleeding Heart ▲✚ — accepting pain of broken relationships in family of origin
Blue Elf Viola ❖ — release of anger and frustration

● BACH — ■ MASTER'S — ▲ FES — ▼ GREEN HOPE — ◆ AUSTRALIAN BUSH
❭ LIVING/AUSTRALIA — ❖ ALASKAN — ✚ PEGASUS — ✪ PERELANDRA

Buttercup ▲✚ — tendency to still see self in persona of small, vulnerable child

California Wild Rose ▲✚ — accepting pain of childhood, moving past victim role

Calla Lily ▲✚ — healing mixed messages about sexual identity from childhood

Canyon Dudleya ▲ — acting out or dramatizing childhood trauma in adult life

Centaury ● — compulsion to serve parents, family members, parent-like figures

Cerato ●✚ — trusting inner knowing which was invalidated by parents

Cherry Plum ●✚ — fear that childlike spontaneity will lead to loss of control

Chicory ●✚ — behaving in childish way to get attention

Cotton Grass ✤ — moving focus of inner child from pain to healing

Dogwood ▲ — childhood abuse/neglect which disconnects from sense of beauty

Echinacea ▲✚ — reclaiming one's integrity/dignity despite prior abuse/trauma

Elm ●✚ — overwhelm due to premature assuming of adult responsibilities

Evening Primrose ▲ — accepting that one was rejected/unwanted in utero/at birth

Fairy Lantern ▲ — attachment to childlike identity as a way of pleasing elders

Forget-Me-Not ▲✚✤ — getting back in touch with original innocence

Fuchsia ▲ — emotional catharsis

Golden Ear Drops ▲ — contacting/releasing painful childhood memories

Goldenrod ▲▼✚ — establishing identity apart from family structure

Grove Sandwort ✤ — strengthening bonds of communication with earth mother

Holly ●✚ — childhood abuse, conditional love or sibling rivalry, crippling heart

Iris ▲ — contacting creativity which may have been suppressed in childhood

Lady's Slipper ▲✤ — directing healing energy to the inner child

Larch ●✚ — suppression of childlike spontaneity

Mariposa Lily ▲ — healing core relationship with one's mother

Milkweed ▲✚ — unconscious desire to merge with parents

Northern Lady's Slipper ❖ — healing core traumas

Old Maid ✚ — acceptance/forgiveness of one's parents

Onion ▲✚ — supports inner child processing

Oregon Grape ▲ — overcoming childhood conditioning of expecting the worst

Pine ● — blaming self for family dysfunction

Pink Monkeyflower ▲ — sense of shame from childhood abuse

Pink Yarrow ▲ — coped as child by being a container of emotional refuse of family

Pretty Face ▲ — ugly duckling/black sheep of the family

Purple Monkeyflower ▲ — overemphasis on "fearing God" in childhood

Red Clover ▲▼ — reacts rather than acts in family crisis, prone to hysteria/panic

Rosemary ▲▼✚ — for those who learned to disembody from abuse

Scarlet Monkeyflower ▲ — contact/acknowledge anger from childhood

Self-Heal ▲ — moving beyond victim role, responsibility for own healing

Shooting Star ▲✚❖ — traumatic or extremely disturbed birthing situation

Sunflower ▲▼✚❖ — disturbed relationship with father

Willow ●✚ — releasing blame and bitterness for childhood pain

Yerba Santa ▲✚ — unclaimed grief from childhood stored in heart

Zinnia ▲▼✚✪ — to encourage exuberance, joyful involvement in life

Inner Strength

Allamanda ✚ — inner strength, inner confidence

Aspen ● — inner strength from the spiritual world

Blue China Orchid ◗ — to strengthen will and take back control of self

Centaury ● — serving others from inner strength

Cerato ●✚ — increases inner strength

Goddess Grasstree ◗ — metamorphosis to inner strength

Illawara FlameTree ◆ — self approval, self-reliance, inner strength

Fawn Lily ▲ — inner strength to face the world

Maple (Sugar) ✚ — deep inner strength and balance

Pink Fairy Orchid ◗ — to carry own peace and be discerning

● BACH — ■ MASTER'S — ▲ FES — ▼ GREEN HOPE — ◆ AUSTRALIAN BUSH
◗ LIVING/AUSTRALIA — ❖ ALASKAN — ✚ PEGASUS — ✪ PERELANDRA

Snake Vine ❱ — confidence/appreciation of achievements amidst malice/doubt

Thistle ▼ — to access inner strength

Wooly Banksia ❱ — desire to pursue ideals/goals when struggle seems too much

Insecurity

Aspen ● — anxiety about the unknown and the future

Baby Blue Eyes ▲▼ — mistrust from abandonment/estrangement from father

Calla Lily ▲✚ — uncertainty and confusion about sexual identity

Dog Rose ◆ — fearful, shy, apprehensive of others, niggling fears

Evening Primrose ▲ — unconscious belief that one is unwanted and unloved

Fairy Lantern ▲ — instability/insecurity in relationships

Garlic ▲✚ — psychic fears which weaken vitality, thus producing insecurity

Golden Yarrow ▲ — fear of performance or social contact, hypersensitivity

Goldenrod ▲▼✚ — socially insecure, trying to measure up to others' standards

Happy Wanderer ❱ — essence inspires a realization of self reliance/determination

Mallow ▲▼✚ — social insecurities that hinder ability to make friends

Mimulus ●✚ — overly fearful, timid, fretful

Persimmon ▲✚ — low self-esteem, sexual inhibitions, lack of proper sexual identity

Pink Monkeyflower ▲ — insecurity characterized by shame/defensiveness

Pretty Face ▲ — social insecurity due to over-concern about appearance

Rosemary ▲▼✚ — not feeling safe in physical body

St. John's Wort ▲▼✚ — insecure sleeping alone or going to sleep

Star Thistle ▲ — lack of feeling secure in self, tendency to accumulate possessions

Strawberry ■▲✚ — feeling unworthy, undeserving, irresponsible

Tall Mulla Mulla ◆ — ill at ease, fear of circulating and mixing

---

● BACH — ■ MASTER'S — ▲ FES — ▼ GREEN HOPE — ◆ AUSTRALIAN BUSH
❱ LIVING/AUSTRALIA — ✤ ALASKAN — ✚ PEGASUS — ✪ PERELANDRA

Insensitivity

Aloe Vera ▲▼✚ — lack of sensitivity from a burned out feeling

Calendula ▲▼✚ — difficulty listening

Flannel Flower ◆ — gentleness, sensitivity in touching, joy, trust, sensuality

Green Bog Orchid ✤ — sensitivity through release of pain/fear held deep in heart

Kangaroo Paw ◆ — unaware of appropriate social behavior

Orange Leschenaultia ◗ — brings in touch with softness of life, empathy re-emerges

Peach ■▲✚ — inability to relate to others' realities

Raspberry ■✚ — kindness, compassion, empathy

Red and Green Kangaroo Paw ◗ — in touch with loved ones, promoting sensitivity

Red Helmet Orchid ◆ — helps father/child bonding, sensitivity, respect

Red Leschenaultia ◗ — discourages harshness or hard-heartedness

Yellow Star Tulip ▲ — compassionate presence

Zucchini ▲▼✚✪ — increases sensitivity in men

Insight

Aconite ✚ — insight, balancing lower and higher self

Angelica ▲▼✚ — insight into the spiritual world

Blackberry ■▲▼✚ — putting ideas into action, overcoming inertia

Black-Eyed Susan ▲▼◆ — insight into emotions, especially dark or blocked emotions

Bush Iris ◆ — spiritual insight

Chestnut Bud ●✚ — understanding lessons gained from life experiences

Endive ✚ — insight into health

Fuchsia ▲ — awareness/understanding of emotions masked by false emotionality

Hound's Tongue ▲✚ — higher meaning of intellectual ideas/material phenomena

Hyssop ▲▼✚ — insight into behavior

Mugwort ▲✚ — clarity about dream life/events outside rational consciousness

Queen Anne's Lace ▲▼✚ — integration of sight with sensitivity/clairvoyance

Rosa Beggeriana ✚ — psychic sight/ability to have insight into personal issues

Rosa Escae ✚ — insight and intuition

Sage ▲✚ — insight into meaning of life, wisdom and acceptance

Shasta Daisy ▲ — synthesis of many idea into one whole

Star Tulip ▲✚ — inner knowing from one's own meditative attunement

Tansy ▲✚ — insight and understanding

Yellow Star Tulip ▲ — insight through social interaction, listening skills

Insomnia

Aspen ● — fear of the dark or unknown

Balm-Lemon ✚ — eases insomnia

Basil ▲✚✪ — anxiety, depression, hysteria, indecision, insomnia, and mental fatigue

Black-Eyed Susan ▲▼◆ — insomnia due to troubling thoughts which are repressed

Chamomile ▲✚ — calming hypertension, emotional upset

Chaparral ▲✚ — intense cathartic dreams which trouble psyche, cause fitful sleep

Dill ▲▼✪ — insomnia due to nervous or sensory overwhelm

Lavender ▲✚ — overwrought nerves

Licorice ✚ — calms restlessness

Mugwort ▲✚ — disturbed sleep due to overactive dream life

Red Chestnut ●✚ — insomnia due to excessive worry and concern about others

St. John's Wort ▲▼✚ — disturbed, fearful dreams, fear of the dark/sleep

Sandalwood ✚ — fear of heights, insomnia, depression, and stress

White Chestnut ● — insomnia caused by repetitive, obsessive thoughts

Valerian ▲✚ — exhaustion, disturbed sleep, tension, stress

Ylang Ylang ✚ — calms anger, frustration, stress, depression, insomnia

Inspiration

Blackberry ■▲▼✚ — putting ideas into action, overcoming inertia

Blue Flag Iris ▼✚ — inspires artistic creativity

Bougainvillaea ▼✚ — higher inspiration, enthusiasm and purposefulness

Cherry ■✚ — inspiration to others, optimistic, positive

Chokecherry ✚ — clears out darkness and clarifies motivations

Cosmos ▲▼✚ — ability to articulate higher inspiration in thoughts/speech

Ginger ▲▼✚ — sterility in creativity, for an artist needing inspiration and new ideas

Goldenrod ▲▼✚ — spiritual inspiration

Grape ■ — realization of the inner source of love

Gum Plant ▲✚ — inspirational writing

Heliconia ✚ — gathering ideas, initiating them, accepting results, making changes

Hound's Tongue ▲✚ — higher meaning of intellectual ideas/material phenomena

Indian Paintbrush ▲✚ — to ground inspired/creative activity, especially when overtaxed

Iris ▲ — to spark inspired thinking and creative activity

Mugwort ▲✚ — to balance/integrate psychic forces with inspired thought

Parakeelya ◗ — to be the inspired worker who can enjoy belonging to the group

Past Life Orchid ✚ — self-knowledge, deep understanding, inspiration, integration

Plum Tree ✚ — manifests inspiration and new ideas

Red Beak Orchid ◗ — renews energy and inspiration

Shasta Daisy ▲ — synthesis of many idea into one whole

Silk Tree ✚ — promotes a transcendental perspective, inspiration, self-integration

Star Tulip ▲✚ — receptivity to spiritual information

Tundra Rose ❖ — opening to inspiration

Instability

Barley ✚ — anger, aggression, and instability

Belladonna ✚ — spiritual instability

Chamomile ▲✚ — emotional instability

Solomon's Seal ✚ — emotional instability, low self-esteem, and over-inquisitiveness

Tomato ■▼✚✪ — defensiveness, instability

Instinctual Self

Alpine Lily ▲ — alienation from feminine sexuality and sexual organs

---

● BACH — ■ MASTER'S — ▲ FES — ▼ GREEN HOPE — ◆ AUSTRALIAN BUSH
◗ LIVING/AUSTRALIA — ❖ ALASKAN — ✚ PEGASUS — ✪ PERELANDRA

California Pitcher Plant ▲✚ — fear of the instinctual aspects of the self

Easter Lily ▲✚ — conflict about sexuality, feeling it is impure or "lower"

Edelweiss ✚ — activates original instinctive or intuitive responses

Hibiscus ▲ — experiencing sexuality as a positive expression of the body

Manzanita ▲✚ — aversion to the physical body

Noni ▲ — awakening instincts of nurturing, caring and love

Pomegranate ▲▼✚ — conflicts about feminine procreative instinct

Queen Anne's Lace ▲▼✚ — integration of psychic and sexual energies

Scarlet Monkeyflower ▲ — fear of instincts relating to power, survival, anger

Snapdragon ▲▼✚ — contacting core feelings of anger/sexuality when aggressive

Sticky Monkeyflower ▲ — difficulty integrating sexual instincts with heart

Tiger Lily ▲✚ — transmuting hostile or aggressive tendencies

Trillium ▲▼✚ — transforming lower instincts of greed or lust for power

Intellect

Bloodroot ▲▼✚ — single point of focus, concentration, and meditation

Cosmos ▲▼✚ — overly wordy, rapid/rambling speech

Hound's Tongue ▲✚ — sense-bound or materialistic ideas

Isopogon ◆ — retrieval of forgotten skills

Jerusalem Artichoke ✚ — stimulates intellect, stabilizes mood

Lemon ▲▼✚ — clarity of thought

Nasturtium ▲▼✚✪ — dry intellect which suppresses vitality

Ragweed-Ambrosia ✚ — dry intellectual becomes more emotional

Rose - Buff Beauty ✚ — stimulates intellect to better deal with city pressures

Rosa Cinnamomea ✚ — balancing philosophical issues

Shasta Daisy ▲ — to balance analytic thinking with holistic overview

Zinnia ▲▼✚✪ — overly serious or intellectual, need to lighten up

Intimacy

Avocado ■▲▼✚ — brings forward feelings of intimacy

Baby Blue Eyes ▲▼ — restoration of childlike innocence and trust

● BACH — ■ MASTER'S — ▲ FES — ▼ GREEN HOPE — ◆ AUSTRALIAN BUSH
◗ LIVING/AUSTRALIA — ✤ ALASKAN — ✚ PEGASUS — ✪ PERELANDRA

Basil ▲✚❂ — polarizing physical intimacy/sexual desire with spiritual ideals

Calendula ▲▼✚ — expressing warmth, intimacy and nurturing feelings with words

Evening Primrose ▲ — can't express intimacy from past rejection, cold/distant

Fawn Lily ▲ — to develop intimate/warm contact with others, aloofness

Golden Yarrow ▲ — to develop social contact/rapport, while remaining sensitive

Grape ■ — loving without condition, demand or expectation

Hibiscus ▲ — experiencing sexuality as a positive expression of the body

Holly Thorn ✚ — allows intimacy and the expression of our truth and creativity

Mallow ▲▼✚ — greater social warmth, ability to sustain relationships, friendships

Mariposa Lily ▲ — deprived of mother/parenting resulting in coldness in the soul

Peony ▲✚ — fear of intimacy

Pink Monkeyflower ▲ — allowing feelings to flow through heart more easily

Pink Yarrow ▲ — establishing intimacy without inappropriate merging

Poison Ivy ▲✚ — fear physical intimacy, are generally anxious or irritable

Poison Oak ▲ — fear of making contact, especially of being touched, fear of enmeshment

Shooting Star ▲✚❖ — profound alienation from human contact and warmth

Star Tulip ▲✚ — softness and receptivity, soul gentleness

Sticky Monkeyflower ▲ — conflict/fear of intimacy, of being vulnerable

Violet ▲ — fear of losing individuality in group, tendency to shyness/retreat

Water Violet ●✚ — inability to establish intimate contact from disdain/superiority

Wisteria ◆ — fulfillment and enjoyment of sexuality

Yellow Star Tulip ▲ — to develop and establish empathetic contact

Intolerance

Beech ●✚ — hard, judgemental, demanding, unrealistic perfectionism

Belladonna ✚ — intolerance, inappropriate strictness, constant anger

Date ■ — judgemental, critical, intolerant

Green Rose ✚❱ — maintaining disciplines and healthy habits

Impatiens ●✚ — impatience, irritation, tension, intolerance

Slender Rice Flower ◆ — racism formed from personal experience, narrow minded

Vervain ●✚ — intense and overbearing influence on others

Yellow and Green Kangaroo Paw ❱ — for those frustrated by mistakes of others

Yellow Leschenaultia ❱ — to stimulate open-mindedness

Yellow Star Tulip ▲ — to develop and establish empathetic contact

Introversion

Bee Balm ✚ — for a clearer expression of one's problems

Cinnamon ✚ — for a clearer expression of one's feelings

Cosmos ▲▼✚ — for introverted, shy, procrastinating people

Fawn Lily ▲ — to develop intimate/warm contact with others

Five Corners ◆ — love and acceptance of self, celebration of own beauty

Frangipani ✚ — for introverts and nervous people

Fringed Lily Twiner ❱ — loss of balanced perspective leading to introversion

Mallow ▲▼✚ — greater social warmth, ability to sustain relationships, friendships

Rosa California ✚ — for introverts, opens heart chakra

Rosa Fendleri Woodsii ✚ — overcomes acute introversion, fear of meeting people

Rosemary ▲▼✚ — lack of physical warmth and presence

Sensitive Plant ✚ — extremely shy and withdrawn or introverted

Sweet Woodruff ✚ — introverts learn to communicate

Tall Mulla Mulla ◆ — ill at ease, fear of circulating and mixing, loner

White Spider Orchid ❱ — brings love and caring to darkest corners of the world

---

● BACH — ■ MASTER'S — ▲ FES — ▼ GREEN HOPE — ◆ AUSTRALIAN BUSH
❱ LIVING/AUSTRALIA — ✿ ALASKAN — ✚ PEGASUS — ✪ PERELANDRA

Intuition

Bush Fuchsia ◆ — feeling unbalanced, not trusting intuition

Cerato ●✚ — trusting inner knowing

Daffodil ▲▼✚ — deepens communication with entire self

Daisy ✚ — enhancing clear link to intuition, developing connection to higher mind

Edelweiss ✚ — activates original instinctive or intuitive responses

Eggplant ▼✚ — deep knowing, intuition

Eyebright ✚ — for healers/practitioners to better perceive condition of client

Fig ■▲✚ — self-limiting

Fireweed ▲❖✚ — clarity in inner knowing and intuition

Four Leaf Clover ✚ — increases practical, logical thinking and intuition

French Marigold ▼ — increases intuitive understanding of information

Gum Plant ▲✚ — increases intuition

Lamb's Quarters ❖ — balancing the intuitive with the rational

Mignonette ▼ — encourages intuition

Moschatel ❖ — opens intuition with the plant kingdom

Pansy ▲✚ — increases intuitive faculties and strengthens mental functioning

Prayer Plant ✚ — develops internal dialogue and intuition

Rhubarb ✚ — balance between analytical and intuitive

Rosa Beggeriana ✚ — intuition increases

Rosa Damascena Versicolor ✚ — telepathy/intuitive processes better understood

Rosa Escae ✚ — insight and intuition

Skullcap ✚ — increases awareness of one's intuitive response to others

Sunflower ▲▼✚❖ — clarifies intuition

Viburnum ✚ — strengthens psychic abilities

Wake Robin ✚ — enhances ability to make intuitive decisions

White Spruce ❖ — balance of logic and intuition

Involvement

California Wild Rose ▲✚ — enthusiastic involvement in life

Cape Honeysuckle ✚ — balancing grief, loneliness, or other difficult emotion states

---

● BACH — ■ MASTER'S — ▲ FES — ▼ GREEN HOPE — ◆ AUSTRALIAN BUSH
◗ LIVING/AUSTRALIA — ❖ ALASKAN — ✚ PEGASUS — ✪ PERELANDRA

Evening Primrose ▲ — enhanced emotional presence, resolving childhood trauma

Fawn Lily ▲ — to develop intimate/warm contact with others

Forget-Me-Not ▲✚✤ — loneliness and feelings of spiritual isolation

Golden Yarrow ▲ — greater involvement in life/public affairs, despite sensitivity

Gooseberry ✚ — fear of getting involved

Green Rose ✚◗ — to move forward

Holly Thorn ✚ — withholding oneself, lack of involvement

Hornbeam ● — involvement in the tasks of life, especially when tired for no reason

Love-Lies-Bleeding ▲ — profound melancholia and anguish, especially private suffering

Mallow ▲▼✚ — greater social warmth, ability to sustain relationships, friendships

Mariposa Lily ▲ — emotional connection with others, feeling separate and unloved

Peach ■▲✚ — concern for welfare of others, empathy, nurturance

Pink Mulla Mulla ◆ — forgiveness, trusting, opening up

Shooting Star ▲✚✤ — feeling at home, overcoming deep-seated alienation

Single Delight ✤ — feelings of isolation

Sweet Pea ▲✚ — finding roots in community life, developing sense of place

Tall Mulla Mulla ◆ — ill at ease, fear of circulating and mixing, loner

Tall Yellow Top ◆ — feeling lonely, isolated

Trillium ▲▼✚ — involvement with others for the greater social good

Veronica ◗ — feel misunderstood, lonely and isolated

Violet ▲ — fear of losing individuality in group, tendency to shyness/retreat

Water Violet ●✚ — sharing, overcoming aloofness or pride

Irrational Behavior

Aspen ● — anxiety about the unknown and the future

Onion ▲✚ — releases toxic emotions and mental barriers

Scarlet Monkeyflower ▲ — explosive emotions from powerlessness, suppressed rage

---

● BACH — ■ MASTER'S — ▲ FES — ▼ GREEN HOPE — ◆ AUSTRALIAN BUSH
◗ LIVING/AUSTRALIA — ✤ ALASKAN — ✚ PEGASUS — ✪ PERELANDRA

Irritability

Beech ●✚ — hard, judgemental, demanding, unrealistic perfectionism
Chamomile ▲✚ — calming hypertension, emotional upset
Chicory ●✚ — needing and demanding personal attention
Crab Apple ●▼✚ — disgust with imperfection and impurities
Date ■ — judgemental, critical, intolerant
Dill ▲▼✪ — irritability due to nervous or sensory overwhelm
Impatiens ●✚ — impatience, irritation, tension, intolerance
Indian Pink ▲✚ — feeling upset by frenetic activity
Lavender ▲✚ — overwrought nerves
Pink Yarrow ▲ — easily upset by emotional disturbance in others
Poison Ivy ▲✚ — fear physical intimacy, is generally anxious or irritable
Poison Oak ▲ — projecting hostility to keep others away
Snapdragon ▲▼✚ — easily set off to make verbal attacks, snapping
Willow ●✚ — resentment, blame of others, hatred over time turning to bitterness
Yarrow ▲ — vulnerability to disturbances in the environment

Isolation (see Involvement)

Jealousy

Apple ■▲✚ — anger, jealousy and fear
Grape ■ — envy, greed, lust, jealousy
Holly ●✚ — hostility toward others out of jealousy, rivalry, etc
Mountain Devil ◆ — hatred, jealousy, holding grudges, suspicion
Pretty Face ▲ — envious of the physical appearance of others
Trillium ▲▼✚ — coveting the power/possessions of others, greed

Joy

Alpine Mint Bush ◆ — revitalization, joy, renewal
Angel's Trumpet ▲✚ — acceptance of death as a joyous transition
Apple ■▲✚ — hope, motivation, a positive outlook
Baby Blue Eyes ▲▼ — restoration of childlike innocence and trust
Bluebell ◆ — opens the heart, joy, sharing
Borage ▲▼✚ — uplifts the heart, dispels gloom and sorrow, gives courage

---

● BACH — ■ MASTER'S — ▲ FES — ▼ GREEN HOPE — ◆ AUSTRALIAN BUSH
◗ LIVING/AUSTRALIA — ✤ ALASKAN — ✚ PEGASUS — ✪ PERELANDRA

Calla Lily ▲✚ — returning a sense of joy and freedom

Calypso Orchid ✚ — joy, playfulness, communion, bonding

Chiming Bells ❖ — joy in physical existence

Corn ■▲▼✚✪ — energy, joy, taking initiative

Flannel Flower ◆ — gentleness, sensitivity in touching, joy, trust, sensuality

Holly ●✚ — ability to feel happiness for others, joy in accomplishments of others

Hornbeam ● — listless for no apparent reason

Impatiens ●✚ — taking the time to experience the joy of life

Larkspur ▲✚ — providing leadership with joy, charisma

Little Flannel Flower ◆ — playfulness, joyful, ability to have fun, spontaneity

Mustard ●✚ — transforming depression into quiet, balanced joy

Orange ■ — cultivating an inner smile

Peach ■▲✚ — able to know the joy of love

Pink Everlasting ◗ — restoring milk of human kindness to hearts

Plantain ▲ — restores joy and spontaneity

Red and Green Kangaroo Paw ◗ — allowing time for the little joys in life

Rhododendron ✚ — warmth, consolation and a sense of joy

Spinach ■ — childlike joy, playfulness, freedom

Tundra Rose ❖ — joy in the fulfillment of life's challenges

Zinnia ▲▼✚✪ — to encourage exuberance, joyful involvement in life

Judgement

Banana ■▲▼✚ — clouded judgement

Beech ●✚ — hard, judgemental, demanding, unrealistic perfectionism

Blackberry ■▲▼✚ — fault finding nature

Cerato ●✚ — ability to judge for oneself rather than relying on others

Date ■ — judgemental, critical, intolerant

Fig ■▲✚ — judgemental of self

Milkmaids ✚ — critical of self and others

Mullein ▲✚ — developing inner values and moral choices

Pine ● — severe self-judgement, guilt and self-blame

Pineapple ■✚ — judging self in comparison to others

Queen Anne's Lace ▲▼✚ — clarity in psychic perception and judgement

Scleranthus ●✚ — forming clear judgements instead of vacillating

● BACH — ■ MASTER'S — ▲ FES — ▼ GREEN HOPE — ◆ AUSTRALIAN BUSH
◗ LIVING/AUSTRALIA — ❖ ALASKAN — ✚ PEGASUS — ✪ PERELANDRA

Sphagnum Moss ❖ — inappropriate judgement and criticism
Yellow Cowslip Orchid ◆ — critical, judgemental, bureaucratic

Kindness

Blackberry ■▲▼✚ — seeing goodness within self and others
Peach ■▲✚ — concern for welfare of others, empathy, nurturance
Pink Everlasting ◗ — restoring milk of human kindness to hearts
Raspberry ■✚ — kindness, compassion, empathy

Laughter

Ice Plant ▼ — joy, bliss and laughter
Little Flannel Flower ◆ — playfulness, joyful, ability to have fun, spontaneity
Zinnia ▲▼✚✪ — to encourage exuberance, joyful involvement in life

Laziness

Corn ■▲▼✚✪ — sluggishness, dragging one's feet, lethargy
Kapok Bush ◆ — resignation, easily discouraged, apathy
Peppermint ▲✚ — dull or sluggish, especially mental lethargy
Red Feather Flower ◗ — problems with energy and attitude leading to laziness
Sycamore ✚ — profound fatigue and exhaustion
Veronica ◗ — laziness, weakness in individuality

Leadership

Elm ●✚ — overly perfectionist or anxious leadership
Jacob's Ladder ❖✚ — problems making decisions in leadership position
Lady's Slipper ▲❖ — blocked leadership potential, often with nervous exhaustion
Larkspur ▲✚ — providing leadership with joy, charisma
Mountain Pride ▲✚ — warrior-like courageous leadership, ability to face adversity
Oak ●✚ — never-ceasing effort in spite of poor health or reduced forces
One-Sided Bottlebrush ◗ — feeling unsupported/overwhelmed in leadership position
Red Clover ▲▼ — leadership in crisis situations, keeping calm amidst panic

---

● BACH — ■ MASTER'S — ▲ FES — ▼ GREEN HOPE — ◆ AUSTRALIAN BUSH
◗ LIVING/AUSTRALIA — ❖ ALASKAN — ✚ PEGASUS — ✪ PERELANDRA

Sage ▲✚ — calm, wise leadership, letting go of personal ambition and importance

Sunflower ▲▼✚✣ — radiant individuality, positive influence on others

Tiger Lily ▲✚ — sense of receptivity and cooperation, balancing overaggressiveness

Trumpet Vine ▲✚ — ability to speak out vigorously to the public

Vervain ●✚ — strong leadership which can become overly intense or fanatical

Vine ●✚ — tendency to authoritarian, despotic leadership

Learning Difficulties

Bush Fuchsia ◆ — allows one to integrate information

California Wild Rose ▲✚ — boredom/lack of interest in study material

Chamomile ▲✚ — emotional hyperactivity

Chestnut Bud ●✚ — repeating errors, difficulty learning lessons

Clematis ●✚ — difficulty paying attention in class, daydreaming or fantasizing

Cosmos ▲▼✚ — speech difficulties when mind is overwhelmed

Daisy ✚ — ability to integrate many different thoughts

Gentian ●✚ — giving up when difficulties are encountered

Impatiens ●✚ — can't pay attention, restlessness, unable to focus, hyperactive

Iris ▲ — lacking in creative insight or interest

Isopogon ◆ — retrieval of forgotten skills

Loofa (Lufa) ▲✚ — hyperactivity, defines skin as the space of the physical body

Madia ▲✚ — short attention span, flits from one activity to another

Milkweed ▲✚ — emotional immaturity, leading to learning difficulties

Penstemon ▲✚ — physical/mental handicaps which make learning difficult

Peppermint ▲✚ — stimulating mental capacities, especially when dull or sluggish

Rabbitbrush ▲✚ — mental flexibilty and alertness, handle many different details

Rubber Tree ✚ — for lack of concentration, lethargy, and spaciness

Self-Heal ▲ — confidence when faced with learning difficulties from injury/illness

Trumpet Vine ▲✚ — problems with speech, such as stuttering

Yarrow ▲ — environmental sensitivity which prevents concentration/focus

Yellow Leschenaultia ◗ — learning difficulties in children, adults including autism

Lethargy

Blackberry ■▲▼✚ — putting ideas into action, overcoming inertia

Corn ■▲▼✚✪ — sluggishness, dragging one's feet, lethargy

Cosmos ▲▼✚ — to stimulate mental clarity, especially lively, thoughtful speech

Hornbeam ● — intimidated by the tasks of everyday life

Horseradish ✚ — boredom, lethargy, depression, or hysteria

Peppermint ▲✚ — stimulating mental capacities, especially when dull or sluggish

Red Beak Orchid ◗ — renews energy and inspiration

Robinia ✚ — for the overly lethargic individual

Rubber Tree ✚ — for lack of concentration, lethargy, and spaciness

Sugar Cane ✚ — sharp mood swings, lethargy, and general depression

Sycamore ✚ — profound fatigue and exhaustion

Tansy ▲✚ — procrastinating, lethargic, overly phlegmatic, indecisive

Tea Plant ✚ — overcoming mental lethargy, stagnation

Life Direction

Baby Blue Eyes ▲▼ — feeling stymied, cynical, bitter, unable to trust

Blackberry ■▲▼✚ — putting ideas into action, overcoming inertia

Buttercup ▲✚ — feeling the worth of one's life work and vocation

California Wild Rose ▲✚ — accepting/responding to the challenges of life

Chrysanthemum ▲✚ — awareness of own mortality

Corn ■▲▼✚✪ — focus on new life directions

Fairy Lantern ▲ — resolving and releasing the past

Gentian ●✚ — easily discouraged or pessimistic about life's direction

Lady's Slipper ▲✤ — to integrate spiritual purpose with daily work

Larch ●✚ — confidence to follow creative inspiration and life destiny

Pomegranate ▲▼✚ — for women, conflict between family and career

Sage ▲✚ — for advanced stages of life, absorbing life and imparting wisdom

---

● BACH — ■ MASTER'S — ▲ FES — ▼ GREEN HOPE — ◆ AUSTRALIAN BUSH
◗ LIVING/AUSTRALIA — ✤ ALASKAN — ✚ PEGASUS — ✪ PERELANDRA

Sagebrush ▲✚ — periods of inactivity or setback
Scleranthus ●✚ — vacillating between two choices
Shooting Star ▲✚✣ — not feeling part of humanity
Silver Princess ◆ — aimless, despondent, lacking life direction
Sweet Pea ▲✚ — for the constant wanderer or traveler unable to commit
Walnut ●✚ — breaking free from cultural/family influences
Wild Oat ● — confusion about vocation and life destiny

Lightness

Angel Orchid ✚ — lightness, raising energy
Angelica ▲▼✚ — feeling spiritual guidance and enlightenment
Apricot ▲✚ — gaiety and lightness
Borage ▲▼✚ — uplifts the heart, dispels gloom and sorrow, gives courage
Cherry ■✚ — light-hearted
Cosmos ▲▼✚ — mercurial lightness in thought and speech
Daisy ✚ — calm and centered amid intense activity, lightness, presence
Grass of Parnassus ✣ — receiving nourishment from non-visible light
Hound's Tongue ▲✚ — feeling too weighed down
Iris ▲ — ability to catalyze inspired thought, creative activity
Larkspur ▲✚ — joy in leadership, altruistic idealism
Mustard ●✚ — uplifting heavy, depressive emotions into joyful balance
Orange ■ — cultivating an inner smile
Peppermint ▲✚ — lightness in thinking, mental alertness
Pretty Face ▲ — bringing more light and radiance into body, especially face
Queen Anne's Lace ▲▼✚ — uplifted vision, fine-tuned perception
St. John's Wort ▲▼✚ — feeling the strength/protection inner light
Single Delight ✣ — awareness of the omnipresence of light
Yarrow ▲ — bringing more light and strength in aura to overcome vulnerability
Zinnia ▲▼✚✪ — childlike humor when overly somber or leaden

Limitation

Birch ▲✚ — transcend limitations of mind
Bog Blueberry ✣ — unconditional acceptance of abundance

● BACH — ■ MASTER'S — ▲ FES — ▼ GREEN HOPE — ◆ AUSTRALIAN BUSH
❱ LIVING/AUSTRALIA — ✣ ALASKAN — ✚ PEGASUS — ✪ PERELANDRA

Blueberry Pollen ❖ — releasing mental limitations to the experience of abundance

Fig ■▲✚ — self-limiting

Foxglove ▲❖✚ — releasing tension around heart caused by mental limitation

Harebell ❖ — bringing unconditional love through the heart

Indian Paintbrush ▲✚ — release emotional frustrations/feelings of self-limitation

Pineapple ■✚ — ability to draw abundance

Spiderwort ✚ — allows the acceptance of limitations

Sticky Geranium ❖ — going beyond previous levels of self-definition

Listening

Banana ■▲▼✚ — objectivity

Bougainvillaea ▼✚ — self-reflection and inner-listening

Calendula ▲▼✚ — hearing the deeper meaning of another's words

California Poppy ▲▼ — inner listening and self-realization

Cassandra ❖ — listening to the sounds of nature

Date ■ — easy to talk to

Forget-Me-Not ▲✚❖ — connection with spiritual guides/departed souls

French Marigold ▼ — not really in touch with what others or your body says

Heather ●✚ — remaining quiet so others can be heard

Impatiens ●✚ — tendency to interrupt, impatient when others speak

Mullein ▲✚ — hearing inner spiritual guidance, especially in moral decision making

Peach ■▲✚ — concern for welfare of others, empathy, nurturance

Raspberry ■✚ — kindness, compassion, empathy

Quaking Grass ▲✚ — listening to the needs of others in group work

Star Tulip ▲✚ — hearing one's inner voice

Twinflower ❖ — balancing listening and speaking skills

Yellow Star Tulip ▲ — sensing the deeper meaning or message of others

Loneliness

Baby Blue Eyes ▲▼ — excessive detachment, numbness toward life, lack of trust

Bleeding Heart ▲✚ — feeling loss and pain of a relationship which has ended

Cape Honeysuckle ✚ — balancing grief, loneliness, or other difficult emotion states

Chin Cactus ✚ — spiritual loneliness

Curry Leaf Tree ✚ — bringing warmth into those who feel alone in this world

Date ■ — closed, intolerant, irritable

Echinacea ▲✚ — profound sense of devastation making one feel utterly alone/bereft

Elm ●✚ — feeling one is alone in facing an overwhelming task

Evening Primrose ▲ — inability to form committed relationships

Forget-Me-Not ▲✚✤ — to counteract feelings of spiritual isolation

Grape ■ — loneliness, feeling disconnected

Heather ●✚ — seeking social contact by talking excessively about problems

Honeysuckle ●✚ — loneliness expressed as nostalgia

Love-Lies-Bleeding ▲ — profound melancholia and anguish, especially private suffering

Mallow ▲▼✚ — overcoming social barriers, developing trust and warmth

Mustard ●✚ — loneliness and isolation from depression and withdrawal

Nicotiana ▲ — appearing solitary or independent but unable to express feelings

Oregon Grape ▲ — feeling cut off from others from paranoid feelings

Parakeelya ◗ — loneliness from lack of appreciation

Peach ■▲✚ — inability to receive love

Pink Monkeyflower ▲ — not expressing intimate feelings from fear of rejection

Sticky Monkeyflower ▲ — conflict/fear of intimacy, of being vulnerable

Sweet Chestnut ●✚ — existential loneliness and despair

Sweet Pea ▲✚ — feeling cut off from community or family ties

Tall Yellow Top ◆ — feeling lonely, isolated

Veronica ◗ — feel misunderstood, lonely and isolated

Violet ▲ — shy about opening to others in a group

Love

Angelica ▲▼✚ — feeling the love and care of spiritual beings

● BACH — ■ MASTER'S — ▲ FES — ▼ GREEN HOPE — ◆ AUSTRALIAN BUSH
◗ LIVING/AUSTRALIA — ✤ ALASKAN — ✚ PEGASUS — ✪ PERELANDRA

Baby Blue Eyes ▲▼ — opening heart to spiritual presence, despite harsh experiences

Black Kangaroo Paw ❱ — forgiveness/love

Bleeding Heart ▲✚ — freedom in love, overcoming unhealthy attachments

California Wild Rose ▲✚ — love as an antidote to apathy

Calla Lily ▲✚ — expressing a greater and deeper sense of love

Celosia ✚ — ability to receive love from others

Chicory ●✚ — selflessness in expressing love

Daffodil ▲▼✚ — replaces depression/low self-worth with love and trust

Fawn Lily ▲ — to develop intimate/warm contact with others

Five Corners ◆ — love and acceptance of self, celebration of own beauty

Forget-Me-Not ▲✚❖ — understanding deeper meaning of relationships

Grape ■ — loving without condition, demand or expectation

Harebell ❖ — bringing unconditional love through the heart

Hawthorne ✚ — cleanses the heart of negativity

Heart Orchid ✚ — heart energy, love, endless love

Holly ●✚ — compassionate understanding of others

Holly Thorn ✚ — opening heart to love

Indian Pipe ✚ — receptivity to a higher love vibration

Love-Lies-Bleeding ▲ — understanding of love through suffering/sacrifice

Love Orchid ✚ — heart opening, love energy, healing

Mariposa Lily ▲ — receptivity to human love, maternal nurturing

Mauve Melaleuca ❱ — the realization that idealism about love is important

Meadow Sweet ▼ — unconditional love, innate self worth

Milkmaids ✚ — sweetness, love and acceptance of self

Mountain Devil ◆ — unconditional love, forgiveness, happiness, inner peace

Noni ▲ — awakening instincts of nurturing, caring and love

Peach ■▲✚ — inability to receive love

Philotheca ◆ — ability to accept praise, acknowledgement and love

Pink Everlasting ❱ — restoring milk of human kindness to hearts

Pink Monkeyflower ▲ — -not expressing intimate feelings from fear of rejection

Pink Tecoma ▼ — the vibration of love, comfort, security

● BACH — ■ MASTER'S — ▲ FES — ▼ GREEN HOPE — ◆ AUSTRALIAN BUSH
❱ LIVING/AUSTRALIA — ❖ ALASKAN — ✚ PEGASUS — ✪ PERELANDRA

Pink Yarrow ▲ — distinguishing love/compassion from sympathetic merging

Prickly Poppy ✚ — increased ability to love in the face of various obstacles

Rosa Centifolia Cristata ✚ — uniting emotions, universal love within consciousness

Rosa Horrida ✚ — universal love

Rosa Macrophylla ✚ — greater love

Rough Bluebell ◆ — compassion, release of inherent love vibration, sensitivity

Self-Heal ▲ — love of self

Tuberose ✚ — opens the heart to receive love and happiness

Tundra Rose ❖ — love of life

Yellow Star Tulip ▲ — to develop compassionate understanding for others needs

Lower Self

Alpine Lily ▲ — perception/unconscious belief female body is lower or inferior

Basil ▲✚❍ — polarizing physical intimacy/sexual desire with spiritual ideals

Black-Eyed Susan ▲▼◆ — insight into inner darkness or hidden aspects of self

California Pitcher Plant ▲✚ — fear of the instinctual aspects of the Self

Chrysanthemum ▲✚ — over-identification with earthly life and persona

Easter Lily ▲✚ — conflict about sexuality, feeling it is impure or "lower"

Fuchsia ▲ — emotional repression, inability to express genuine deep feelings

Hibiscus ▲ — integration of soul warmth and sexual passion

Lotus ▲✚ — spiritual pride which disowns lower energy centers

Monkshood ▲✚❖ — integrates higher and lower self

Nicotiana ▲ — excessive need to ground or armor oneself

Pine ● — severe self-judgement, guilt and self-blame

Queen Anne's Lace ▲▼✚ — to integrate emotions, sexuality with psychic life

Scarlet Monkeyflower ▲ — transforming anger, powerful emotions

Snapdragon ▲▼✚ — libido misplaced as verbal hostility and aggression

Tiger Lily ▲✚ — transmuting hostility and aggressiveness
Trillium ▲▼✚ — coveting the power/possessions of others, greed
Vine ●✚ — tendency to use will to control others

Male/Female Balance

Balga (Blackboy) ◗ — maturing of the male principle within
Chives ▼✪ — awareness of internal masculine and feminine energies
Green Fairy Orchid ✤ — balancing male and female energies in the heart
Macrozamia ◗ — balance to all aspects of male/female
Mullein ▲✚ — smoothes the rough edges of male/female duality
Rattlesnake Plantain Orchid ✚ — men: aggression, women: male/female balance
Red Ginger ✚ — understanding/acceptance of male/female balance
Sitka Spruce Pollen ✤ — balancing power and gentleness in men and women
Sunflower ▲▼✚✤ — strengthening flow of masculine energy in men and women

Manic Depression

Chamomile ▲✚ — emotional hyperactivity
Mustard ●✚ — transforming depression into quiet, balanced joy
Peach Flowered Tea Tree ◆ — mood swings
Periwinkle ✚ — lifting the veil of depression

Manifestation

Aspen ● — inaction due to fear of taking risks, especially anxiety about the unknown
Blackberry ■▲▼✚ — putting ideas into action, overcoming inertia
Blueberry Pollen ✤ — releasing mental limitations to the experience of abundance
Bog Blueberry ✤ — unconditional acceptance of abundance
Borage ▲▼✚ — uplifts the heart, dispels gloom and sorrow, gives courage
Buttercup ▲✚ — feeling vocation/contribution does not count
California Wild Rose ▲✚ — listless and apathetic attitude
Cayenne ▲✚ — cutting through stagnation or indecision

● BACH — ■ MASTER'S — ▲ FES — ▼ GREEN HOPE — ◆ AUSTRALIAN BUSH
◗ LIVING/AUSTRALIA — ✤ ALASKAN — ✚ PEGASUS — ✪ PERELANDRA

Centaury ● — overly servile mentality, empowering self to take responsibility

Cerato ●✚ — hesitating or losing momentum, squandering resources

Chestnut Bud ●✚ — repeating errors, difficulty learning lessons

Chicory ●✚ — excessive neediness which impairs ability to manifest

Clematis ●✚ — too floaty and dreamy, insubstantial ideas and plans

Crab Apple ●▼✚ — obsessive concern with perfection which stymies manifestation

Filaree ▲✚ — unable to manifest due to enmeshment in endless details/distractions

Gentian ●✚ — giving up when difficulties are encountered

Golden Yarrow ▲ — stepping out in world/making changes despite inner sensitivity

Gorse ●✚ — pessimistic attitude which impedes ability to see positive outcome

Hornbeam ● — procrastination, feeling too tired to start/continue a project

Horseradish ✚ — forgotten goals or dreams may be rekindled and acted upon

Impatiens ●✚ — impatience, irritation, tension, intolerance

Indian Paintbrush ▲✚ — lacking vitality to be creative

Iris ▲ — ability to catalyze inspired thought, creative activity

Lady's Slipper ▲✣ — feeling estranged from true talents and capabilities

Larch ●✚ — confidence to follow creative inspiration and life destiny

Madia ▲✚ — short attention span, flits from one activity to another

Mountain Pride ▲✚ — courage to take risks, to stand up and speak out

Penstemon ▲✚ — inner strength and fortitude

Pine ● — severe self-judgement, guilt and self-blame

Plum Tree ✚ — manifests inspiration and new ideas

Rosa Corilfolia Froebelii ✚ — manifestation

Rosa Rubrifolia ✚ — ability to manifest love in the world

Scleranthus ●✚ — vacillating

Scotch Broom ▲✚ — overcoming negative or hopeless images of the world

Shasta Daisy ▲ — synthesis of many idea into one whole

Tansy ▲✚ — procrastinating, lethargic, overly phlegmatic, indecisive

Trumpet Vine ▲✚ — healthy self-assertion, especially speaking up/asserting self

---

● BACH — ■ MASTER'S — ▲ FES — ▼ GREEN HOPE — ◆ AUSTRALIAN BUSH
❱ LIVING/AUSTRALIA — ✣ ALASKAN — ✚ PEGASUS — ✪ PERELANDRA

Walnut ●✚ — breaking old ties that hinder

Wild Oat ● — scattered talents and interests

Willow ●✚ — a positive reality from the quality of one's thoughts

Manipulation

Chicory ●✚ — needing and demanding personal attention

Fringed Lily Twiner ◗ — demanding, overconcentration on self

Isopogon ◆ — stubborn and controlling

Pale Sundew ◗ — rapacious, manipulative power playing

Peach ■▲✚ — exploitative nature

Rough Bluebell ◆ — manipulative, exploitative, hurtful

Martyrdom

Canyon Dudleya ▲ — acting out or dramatizing childhood trauma in adult life

Centaury ● — tendency to be doormat for others

Chicory ●✚ — feeling sorry for self, manipulating others to gain sympathy

Elm ●✚ — anxiety about responsibility, feeling weight of world on shoulders

Fig ■▲✚ — fanaticism, over extending self

Heather ●✚ — overabsorption in personal problems or trauma

Larkspur ▲✚ — excessive dutifulness, lack of joy

Love-Lies-Bleeding ▲ — tendency to internalize suffering and pain

Mustard ●✚ — feeling sorry for self because of deep depression

Oak ●✚ — balancing desire to be hero with realistic expectation of strength

Peach ■▲✚ — tendency to smother

Penstemon ▲✚ — perseverance despite hardships such as physical handicaps

Rock Water ● — being overly strict with oneself, self-denial

Sweet Chestnut ●✚ — extreme soul anguish, feeling punished by God

Willow ●✚ — seeing self as a victim, blaming others

Masculine

Agrimony ●✚ — false mask of how a "man should be," not showing true feelings

---

● BACH — ■ MASTER'S — ▲ FES — ▼ GREEN HOPE — ◆ AUSTRALIAN BUSH
◗ LIVING/AUSTRALIA — ✤ ALASKAN — ✚ PEGASUS — ✪ PERELANDRA

Aloe Vera ▲▼✚ — unbalanced work patterns which lead to burnout/exhaustion

Baby Blue Eyes ▲▼ — positive masculine identity combining strength and sensitivity

Balga (Blackboy) ◗ — maturing of the male principle within

Black Cohosh ▲ — tendency to commit sexual abuse or violence

Calendula ▲▼✚ — using words to injure others

Calla Lily ▲✚ — insecurity about male sexual identity

Chives ▼✪ — awareness of internal masculine and feminine energies

Dandelion ▲▼✚❖ — overachiever

Elm ●✚ — anxiety about responsibility, feeling weight of world on shoulders

Fairy Lantern ▲ — healthy maturation, acceptance of adult responsibilities

Golden Ear Drops ▲ — overcoming the cultural bias that men do not cry

Green Fairy Orchid ❖ — balancing male and female energies in the heart

Hound's Tongue ▲✚ — inner, imaginative capacities, especially when preoccupied

Impatiens ●✚ — impatience, irritation, tension, intolerance

Larch ●✚ — developing true self-confidence despite shyness and low self-esteem

Larkspur ▲✚ — providing leadership with joy, charisma

Macrozamia ◗ — balance to all aspects of male/female

Mountain Pride ▲✚ — warrior-like courageous leadership, ability to face adversity

Mullein ▲✚ — smoothes the rough edges of male/female duality

Nicotiana ▲ — appearing solitary or independent but unable to express feelings

Oak ●✚ — balancing desire to be hero with realistic expectation of strength

Oregon Grape ▲ — expecting hostility from others, paranoia

Penstemon ▲✚ — perseverance despite hardships

Pink Monkeyflower ▲ — fear of intimacy/vulnerability, childhood shaming/abuse

Poison Ivy ▲✚ — fear physical intimacy, generally anxious or irritable

Poison Oak ▲ — projecting hostility to keep others away

Rattlesnake Plantain Orchid ✚ — anger and aggression issues

Red Ginger ✚ — understanding/acceptance of male/female balance

Rock Water ● — overly strict ideals for oneself and others, inflexible idealism

Sage ▲✚ — relating to elders or to own higher wisdom

Scarlet Monkeyflower ▲ — transforming anger, powerful emotions

Sitka Spruce Pollen ❖ — balancing power and gentleness in men and women

Star Tulip ▲✚ — softening overly masculine qualities

Sticky Monkeyflower ▲ — conflict/fear of intimacy in sexuality

Sunflower ▲▼✚❖ — expressing own unique sun-like radiant individuality

Tiger Lily ▲✚ — transmuting hostility and aggressiveness

Trillium ▲▼✚ — coveting the power/possessions of others, greed

Vine ●✚ — seeing masculine as dominant/feminine as submissive

Wild Oat ● — finding the inner calling to a line of work

Zinnia ▲▼✚✪ — childlike humor when overly somber or leaden

Massage

Arnica ▲✚ — releasing armoring from parts deeply wounded/traumatized

Calendula ▲▼✚ — bringing overall warmth/healing through touch

Chamomile ▲✚ — soothing/relaxing, especially stomach and solar plexus

Crab Apple ●▼✚ — cleansing when applied topically

Dandelion ▲▼✚❖ — releasing emotional tension stored in musculature

Dogwood ▲ — releasing hardened emotions from abuse

Lavender ▲✚ — relaxing head, neck, shoulders

Manzanita ▲✚ — embodiment

Mugwort ▲✚ — to stimulate warmth/circulation, especially female menses, birth, nursing

Nasturtium ▲▼✚✪ — rejuvenating, refreshing, awakening and vitalizing

Olive ●✚ — bringing renewal when there is extreme fatigue

Pink Monkeyflower ▲ — apply topically for those who feel shame, especially about sex

Pink Yarrow ▲ — emotional merging between client/practitioner

Rosemary ▲▼✚ — lack of physical warmth and presence

St. John's Wort ▲▼✚ — psychic sensitivity, sensitivity to light

Self-Heal ▲ — promoting overall health

Skullcap ✚ — deeper bond with client

Sourgrass ✚ — softening

Star Tulip ▲✚ — opening/sensitizing client/practitioner to the massage

Yarrow ▲ — emotional merging, oversensitivity

Yerba Santa ▲✚ — releasing emotional tension stored in chest

Materialism and Money

Aloe Vera ▲▼✚ — workaholism

Angelica ▲▼✚ — awareness that there is more to life than the material world

Bush Iris ◆ — fear of death, materialism, atheism

California Poppy ▲▼ — compulsion to buy new things

Chrysanthemum ▲✚ — accumulating wealth/power to make life permanent

Crab Apple ●▼✚ — obsessive concern with perfection

Daisy ✚ — recurring problems concerning health, friends, relationships or money

Filaree ▲✚ — obsession with money

Hound's Tongue ▲✚ — seeing the world in materialistic or merely physical ways

Iris ▲ — calculate and value only what is utilitarian, efficient or income producing

Larkspur ▲✚ — altruism and balanced leadership

Money Plant ✚ — worries about money and other personal wants

Pineapple ■✚ — clarity with money issues

Poison Oak ▲ — wanting to conquer the world

Sage ▲✚ — tending to think in terms of short-term profit and private gain

Sagebrush ▲✚ — to discern what is essential and let go of excess

Star Thistle ▲ — lack of feeling secure in Self, tendency to accumulate possessions

Sunflower ▲▼✚✣ — pursuing fame and fortune as exterior forms of recognition

Tiger Lily ▲✚ — overly competitive business drive

Trillium ▲▼✚ — coveting the power/possessions of others, greed

---

● BACH — ■ MASTER'S — ▲ FES — ▼ GREEN HOPE — ◆ AUSTRALIAN BUSH
◗ LIVING/AUSTRALIA — ✣ ALASKAN — ✚ PEGASUS — ◐ PERELANDRA

Vine ●✚ — using money/power as a way of exerting control over others

Yellow Star Tulip ▲ — balancing business life with social and moral awareness

Zinnia ▲▼✚✪ — taking money/business too seriously, need to enjoy life

Meditation

Angel's Trumpet ▲✚ — ability to penetrate to spiritual threshold, especially when dying

Angelica ▲▼✚ — awareness of benevolent spiritual forces

Banyan ✚ — deepens visualization during meditation

Bloodroot ▲▼✚ — single point of focus, concentration, and meditation

Bougainvillaea ▼✚ — to reaffirm our commitment to our spiritual destiny

California Poppy ▲▼ — extreme fascination or involvement with psychic powers

Cantaloupe ✚ — acceptance of higher self

Carnation ✚ — emotional objectivity, the ability to meditate

Cassandra ❖ — quieting the mind

Chamomile ▲✚ — calming, facilitates meditative process

Daffodil ▲▼✚ — deepens communication with entire self

Fawn Lily ▲ — prefers quiet and meditative experience

Forget-Me-Not ▲✚❖ — awareness of spiritual guidance/communication

Hardenbergia Comptonia ✚ — increases meditation and visualization

Horsetail ❖✚ — communication between different levels of consciousness

Hound's Tongue ▲✚ — overly materialistic preventing meditative experience

Hyssop ▲▼✚ — insight into behavior, enhances meditation

Impatiens ●✚ — resistant to taking the time to meditate

Jimson Weed ✚ — stimulates dreams, meditation, alignment to inner guides

Lavender ▲✚ — nervous conditions resulting from unbalanced meditative life

Lotus ▲✚ — enhancing spiritual awareness, deepening meditative experience

Milkweed ▲✚ — use of meditation techniques to blot out/stupefy consciousness

Monkshood ▲✚❖ — integrates higher and lower self

Mugwort ▲✚ — awareness of dreams, conscious control of psychic life

Okra ✚ — very grounding, good for meditation

Paper Birch ❖ — getting in touch with life purpose when faced with decisions

Purple Monkeyflower ▲ — unable to sustain meditation from fear of spiritual world

Purple Nymph Waterlily ◗ — to drink deep from deeper side of one's love nature

Queen Anne's Lace ▲▼✚ — to integrate emotions, sexuality with psychic life

Rosa Centifolia Cristata ✚ — uniting emotions, universal love within consciousness

Rosa Roxburghii ✚ — enhancing meditation and right brain activities

Star Tulip ▲✚ — overcoming blockages to spiritual receptivity, inner listening

Sweetgrass ❖ — cleansing a physical space for meditation or ritual

White Chestnut ● — quieting repetitive or obsessive thoughts, stilling the mind

White Nymph Water Lily ◗ — using higher self to integrate and respond to life

Yellow Boronia ◗ — inspires deep contemplation

Yerba Buena ✚ — acceptance of the nature of God

Memory

Allspice ✚ — promotes memory

Avocado ■▲▼✚ — remembering details

Black-Eyed Susan ▲▼◆ — for recovering memory of past trauma

Buttercup ▲✚ — stimulates mental clarity, memory

Clematis ●✚ — memory and emotional stability increase

Comfrey ▲▼✚✪ — releases nervous tension and improves memory

Coriander ✚ — for poor memory and stress

Eyebright ✚ — weak brain and memory

Fennel ✚ — improves memory of those indecisive, depressed and subject to grief

---

● BACH — ■ MASTER'S — ▲ FES — ▼ GREEN HOPE — ◆ AUSTRALIAN BUSH
◗ LIVING/AUSTRALIA — ❖ ALASKAN — ✚ PEGASUS — ✪ PERELANDRA

Fig ■▲✚ — improves confidence, memory, telepathy and expressive abilities

Flax ✚ — assimilation of information and memory improvement

Forget-Me-Not ▲✚❖ — remembering reality

Frangipani ✚ — good for poor memory possibly due to emotional stress

Gotu Kola ✚ — stimulates memory, including higher memory, for past life recall

Isopogon ◆ — retrieval of forgotten skills

Papaya ▲▼✚ — memory retention

Periwinkle ✚ — clears the memory

Rabbitbrush ▲✚ — mental flexibility and alertness

Rosemary ▲▼✚ — forgetfulness

Menopause

Aloe Vera ▲▼✚ — feeling burnt-out

Alpine Lily ▲ — resistance to bodily changes/fluctuations

Beech ●✚ — moody

Black Cohosh ▲ — anger, rage

Black-Eyed Susan ▲▼◆ — avoidance/denial of menopause symptoms

Borage ▲▼✚ — profound grief

Buttercup ▲✚ — feeling worthless

Canyon Dudleya ▲ — tendency toward hysteria/emotional exaggeration

Crab Apple ●▼✚ — need for body to purify and re-align

Easter Lily ▲✚ — resolving tensions around polarities of sexuality/spirituality

Echinacea ▲✚ — profound sense of devastation making one feel utterly alone/bereft

Fairy Lantern ▲ — inability to release reproductive function

Fuchsia ▲ — strong emotional reactions and bodily symptoms

Hibiscus ▲ — reduced sexual response

Iris ▲ — enabling soul to become more creative

Lavender ▲✚ — frayed nerves or insomnia

Mariposa Lily ▲ — to resolve issues around conception and mothering

Olive ●✚ — bringing renewal when there is extreme fatigue

Pink Yarrow ▲ — excessive emotions

Pomegranate ▲▼✚ — feeling that biological clock is running out

● BACH — ■ MASTER'S — ▲ FES — ▼ GREEN HOPE — ◆ AUSTRALIAN BUSH
❱ LIVING/AUSTRALIA — ❖ ALASKAN — ✚ PEGASUS — ✪ PERELANDRA

Pretty Face ▲ — feeling ugly

Rosemary ▲▼✚ — integrating bodily warmth with soul warmth

Sage ▲✚ — to move to new aspects of the Self

Sagebrush ▲✚ — feelings of emptiness or loss

Scarlet Monkeyflower ▲ — transforming anger, powerful emotions

Self-Heal ▲ — viewing menopause as a healthy transition

Sticky Monkeyflower ▲ — developing new patterns of intimacy

Tiger Lily ▲✚ — eruption of strong animus

Zinnia ▲▼✚✪ — viewing menopause as positive/freeing/celebrating soul joy

Mental Clarity/Chatter/Illness

Blackberry ■▲▼✚ — putting ideas into action, overcoming inertia

Boronia ◆ — obsessive thoughts

Bunchberry ✤ — mental steadfastness and emotional clarity in demanding situations

Buttercup ▲✚ — stimulates mental clarity, memory

Cacao ✚ — promotes increased mental clarity and reduces stress

Cosmos ▲▼✚ — overly active mental state needing greater clarity

Ginseng ✚ — clarity and release of creativity

Grapefruit ▲▼✚ — increased mental clarity

Horseradish ✚ — creates mental clarity

Hound's Tongue ▲✚ — raising sense-bound thinking into spiritual understanding

Iris ▲ — ability to catalyze inspired thought, creative activity

Jacob's Ladder ✤✚ — evolved mental control

Lilac ▲▼✚ — supports mental clarity and muscle relaxation

Madia ▲✚ — focus and concentration

Milkweed ▲✚ — mental impairment, need to re-awaken core identity

Mountain Pennyroyal ▲ — negative thoughts/thinking patterns taken on from others

Nasturtium ▲▼✚✪ — hyperactivity of mental forces leading to extreme fatigue

Papaya ▲▼✚ — clears mental confusion and tension

Peppermint ▲✚ — lightness in thinking, mental alertness

Rabbitbrush ▲✚ — mental flexibility and alertness

Red Hibiscus ▼ — brings harmony to the mind

● BACH — ■ MASTER'S — ▲ FES — ▼ GREEN HOPE — ◆ AUSTRALIAN BUSH
◗ LIVING/AUSTRALIA — ✤ ALASKAN — ✚ PEGASUS — ✪ PERELANDRA

Rosemary ▲▼✚ — forgetfulness

Shasta Daisy ▲ — synthesis of many idea into one whole

W.A. Smokebrush ❱ — difficult concentration, vagueness, feeling muddled

White Chestnut ● — quieting repetitive or obsessive thoughts, stilling the mind

Yerba Santa ▲✚ — profound melancholia

Moderation

Almond ■▲✚ — burning the candle at both ends

Aloe Vera ▲▼✚ — moderation in use of creative and vital forces, overwork

Canyon Dudleya ▲ — letting go of psychic or emotional drama

Chocolate Orchid ✚ — openness, moderation

Dill ▲▼✪ — assimilating many sensory impressions with consciousness

Impatiens ●✚ — moderation of overly impulsive actions

Lavender ▲✚ — overwrought nerves

Morning Glory ▲▼✚ — erratic lifestyle and habits which deplete energy

Vervain ●✚ — moderation in feelings and actions

Mood Swings

Apricot ▲✚ — mood swings linked to hyperglycemia

Barley ✚ — moodiness associated with hypoglycemia

Chamomile ▲✚ — emotional hyperactivity

Cherry ■✚ — moodiness, grumpiness

Kiwi ✚ — eases stress and moodiness

Mustard ●✚ — sudden episodes of depression

Peach Flowered Tea Tree ◆ — mood swings, hypochondria

Rye ✚ — moodiness associated with hypoglycemia

Scleranthus ●✚ — vacillating

Sugar Cane ✚ — sharp mood swings, lethargy, and general depression

Morality

Basil ▲✚✪ — secrecy and deception in sexual behavior

Blackberry ■▲▼✚ — seeing goodness within self and others

California Poppy ▲▼ — distinguish/develop inner moral forces

Cerato ●✚ — overdependence on others for moral values

● BACH — ■ MASTER'S — ▲ FES — ▼ GREEN HOPE — ◆ AUSTRALIAN BUSH
❱ LIVING/AUSTRALIA — ✣ ALASKAN — ✚ PEGASUS — ✪ PERELANDRA

Chestnut Bud ●✛ — learning moral lessons from one's experiences

Crab Apple ●▼✛ — obsessive sense of morality, concern with perfection

Deerbrush ▲ — mixed/hidden motives which undermine moral stance

Easter Lily ▲✛ — alternating between promiscuity and prudishness

Holly ●✛ — compassionate understanding of others

Mountain Pride ▲✛ — becoming a spiritual warrior

Mullein ▲✛ — developing a sense of conscience

Pine ● — extreme moral standards applied to oneself in a punishing way

Purple Monkeyflower ▲ — fear based moral values

Rock Water ● — over rigid sense of morality

Scleranthus ●✛ — inner knowingness to distinguish right from wrong

Star Thistle ▲ — generosity and sharing

Sturt Desert Rose ◆ — to follow inner convictions and morality

Trillium ▲▼✛ — altruistic sacrifice

Vine ●✛ — to encourage respect for the individuality of others

Yellow Star Tulip ▲ — sensitivity to the suffering of others

Mother and Mothering

Alpine Lily ▲ — to experience motherhood as a nurturing, rewarding experience

Beech ●✛ — hard, judgemental, demanding of child

Bottlebrush ▼◆✛ — bonding between mother and child

Buttercup ▲✛ — low self-esteem about identity as mother

Canyon Dudleya ▲ — hysterical tendencies in mothering role

Centaury ● — confusing motherhood with servitude

Cherry Plum ●✛ — feeling that one is beyond limits of coping/out of control

Chicory ●✛ — emotional neediness in mother or child

Corn ■▲▼✛✪ — contacting the archetype of the earth mother

Elm ●✛ — feels despondent/overwhelmed as a mother

Evening Primrose ▲ — rejection of child in utero, disturbance in mother-child bond

Fairy Lantern ▲ — tendency to over mother, keep child overly dependent

Fawn Lily ▲ — integration of spiritual ideals/mundane demands of motherhood

---

● BACH — ■ MASTER'S — ▲ FES — ▼ GREEN HOPE — ◆ AUSTRALIAN BUSH
❯ LIVING/AUSTRALIA — ✤ ALASKAN — ✛ PEGASUS — ✪ PERELANDRA

Forget-Me-Not ▲✚❖ — making a decision to have a child

Goddess Grasstree ◗ — maturing of the female principle in mother

Grove Sandwort ❖ — strengthening bonds of communication with earth mother

Impatiens ●✚ — does things for child, rather than allowing child to learn

Indian Pink ▲✚ — handling simultaneous demands from children and household

Iris ▲ — home and mothering role feels dull or dowdy

Mariposa Lily ▲ — bonding in childhood with mother

Milkweed ▲✚ — unconscious regression/merging with mother/mother figure

Noni ▲ — awakening instincts of nurturing, caring and love

Onion ▲✚ — dissolves trauma of separation between mother and child

Peach ■▲✚ — tendency to smother

Pineapple Weed ❖ — harmony between mothers and children

Pomegranate ▲▼✚ — conflict between family and career

Pumpkin ▼✚ — for integrating femininity in motherhood

Quince ▲✚ — conflicts between power and love in feminine forces

Red Chestnut ●✚ — over-fretful concern about child

Scarlet Monkeyflower ▲ — episodes of uncontrolled rage/power plays with child

Star Thistle ▲ — disturbed bond to mother leading to materialism as security

Star Tulip ▲✚ — developing receptivity as a mother

Yellow Star Tulip ▲ — compassionate attunement to one's child

Zinnia ▲▼✚✪ — seeing motherhood as a grim responsibility

Motivation

Blackberry ■▲▼✚ — putting ideas into action, overcoming inertia

California Wild Rose ▲✚ — enthusiasm and positive involvement in life

Cayenne ▲✚ — cutting through stagnation or indecision

Chokecherry ✚ — clears out darkness and clarifies motivations

Deerbrush ▲ — purity of intention

Forsythia ▲ — motivation towards transformation of old patterns of behavior

Gorse ●✚ — counteracting feelings of hopelessness, especially about personal affairs

---

● BACH — ■ MASTER'S — ▲ FES — ▼ GREEN HOPE — ◆ AUSTRALIAN BUSH
◗ LIVING/AUSTRALIA — ❖ ALASKAN — ✚ PEGASUS — ✪ PERELANDRA

Larch ●✚ — developing true self-confidence

Mountain Pride ▲✚ — warrior-like stamina in the face of adversity/challenge

Neoporteria Cactus ✚ — clarifies/focuses soul's energy for action

Scotch Broom ▲✚ — seeing opportunity for service in spite of difficulties

Silver Princess ◆ — life purpose and direction, motivation

Tansy ▲✚ — procrastinating, lethargic, overly phlegmatic, indecisive

Tundra Rose ❖ — opening to higher sources of motivation, especially in writing

Opium Poppy ❖ — balancing motivation with awareness of accomplishments

Paper Birch ❖ — getting in touch with life purpose when faced with decisions

Nature

Chiming Bells ❖ — awareness of the angelic kingdom in nature

Green Bells of Ireland ▼❖ — opening heart/mind to energy/intelligence in nature

Grove Sandwort ❖ — strengthening bonds of communication with nature

Soapberry ❖ — balancing one's personal power with the power of nature

Spiraea ❖ — awareness of support/nurturing from nature

Neediness

Chicory ●✚ — emotional neediness

Fairy Lantern ▲ — immaturity, helplessness, neediness, childish dependency

Grape ■ — neediness, loneliness, feeling disconnected

Peach ■▲✚ — giving from wholeness rather than neediness

Negativity

Antiseptic Bush ❱ — cleansing of negative influences in environment

Banana ■▲▼✚ — not getting caught up in negativity

Beech ●✚ — seeing others critically, harsh judgement

Blackberry ■▲▼✚ — negativity, pessimism, sarcasm, cynicism

Black Cohosh ▲ — attracting the negativity of others

● BACH — ■ MASTER'S — ▲ FES — ▼ GREEN HOPE — ◆ AUSTRALIAN BUSH
❱ LIVING/AUSTRALIA — ❖ ALASKAN — ✚ PEGASUS — ✪ PERELANDRA

Cherry ■✚ — moodiness, grumpiness

Eggplant ▼✚ — transmutes negativity

Hawthorne ✚ — cleanses the heart of negativity

Holly ●✚ — unable to open heart to love for others

Hollyhock ▲✚ — to release negativity

Mountain Pennyroyal ▲ — negative thoughts/thinking patterns taken on from others

Okra ✚ — ability to see the positive in life and environment

Orange ■ — "might as well get used to it" attitude

Oregon Grape ▲ — expecting hostility from others, paranoia

Petunia St. Germain ▼ — forgiveness and transmutation of all negativity

Pink Yarrow ▲ — sensitivity to negative emotional influences

Plantain ▲ — releases mental blocks and draws off negativity

Poison Ivy ▲✚ — generally anxious or irritable

Poison Oak ▲ — projecting hostility to keep others away

Purple and Red Kangaroo Paw ◗ — circular arguments of blame

Rosa Xanthina ✚ — helps healers remove negativity

Ruta (Rue) ▲✚ — repels negativity

Scarlet Monkeyflower ▲ — strong anger or power plays, often unacknowledged

Sondah ▼ — vibration of light to the heart to remove all negativity

Snapdragon ▲▼✚ — easily set off to make verbal attacks, snapping

Spider Lily ▼✚ — overcoming negative mental states

Ursinia ◗ — engenders positivity and deals effectively with negativity

Willow ●✚ — resentment, blame of others, hatred over time turning to bitterness

Wintergreen ▼✚ — cleanses past life negativity from the aura

Yarrow ▲ — vulnerability to negative influences, especially of mental or psychic nature

Yarrow Special Formula ▲ — negativity in environment from chaos, imbalance

Nervousness

Almond ■▲✚ — nervousness, uneasiness

Aspen ● — acute sensitivity to influences not seen or understood

Banana ■▲▼✚ — clouded judgement, nervousness, quarrelsome nature

Canyon Dudleya ▲ — nervous depletion or excessive excitability

---

● BACH — ■ MASTER'S — ▲ FES — ▼ GREEN HOPE — ◆ AUSTRALIAN BUSH
◗ LIVING/AUSTRALIA — ✣ ALASKAN — ✚ PEGASUS — ✪ PERELANDRA

Chamomile ▲✚ — emotional hyperactivity

Cherry Plum ●✚ — nervousness stemming from fear of losing control

Comfrey ▲▼✚✪ — releases nervous tension and improves memory

Cosmos ▲▼✚ — nervous speech patterns which are too rapid

Feverfew ▲▼ — nervous exhaustion, headaches

French Marigold ▼ — nervousness, jumping at noise

Garlic ▲✚ — psychic fears which weaken vitality

Golden Yarrow ▲ — acute sensitivity, feeling vulnerable

Indian Pink ▲✚ — maintaining centered attitude amidst confusion

Lady's Slipper ▲✿ — prone to nervous idiosyncrasies

Lavender ▲✚ — overwrought nerves

Lettuce ■✚ — "the unruffler"

Mimulus ●✚ — nervousness from everyday fears and worries

Morning Glory ▲▼✚ — nervous problems from overstimulation/chaotic life

Nicotiana ▲ — using smoking/addictive substances to calm or numb

Pink Yarrow ▲ — oversensitivity due to emotional absorption

Purple Monkeyflower ▲ — extreme fear or apprehension from spiritual/occult

Purple Nightshade ✚ — soothes jangled, burned-out nervous states

Rosemary ▲▼✚ — feeling ill at ease in physical body

Valerian ▲✚ — promotes relaxation, contentment

Vervain ●✚ — overly enthusiastic, frayed nerves from overstriving

Waratah ◆ — inability to respond to crisis

Nightmares

Angel's Trumpet ▲✚ — eases nightmares by strengthening the astral body

Aspen ● — hidden fears, nightmares

Chaparral ▲✚ — intense cathartic dreams which trouble psyche, cause fitful sleep

Green Spider Orchid ◆ — nightmares, phobias

Rock Rose ●✚ — deep fear, terror, panic

St. John's Wort ▲▼✚ — fear of the dark, sleep traumas, bedwetting

Scarlet Pimpernel ▲ — recurring nightmares

Snap Pea ▼✪ — clarifies purpose behind dreams and nightmares

Tomato ■▼✚✪ — fear, nightmares, withdrawal

● BACH — ■ MASTER'S — ▲ FES — ▼ GREEN HOPE — ◆ AUSTRALIAN BUSH
◗ LIVING/AUSTRALIA — ✿ ALASKAN — ✚ PEGASUS — ✪ PERELANDRA

Non-Attachment

Angel's Trumpet ▲✚ — acceptance of death/dying process

Bleeding Heart ▲✚ — freedom in love, overcoming unhealthy attachments

Calendula ▲▼✚ — listening to the other, non-interference and receptivity

Chrysanthemum ▲✚ — accepting transitory nature of life without morbidity/despair

Filaree ▲✚ — letting go of common worries, obsessive fastidiousness

Goldenrod ▲▼✚ — detachment from what others think, false persona as a prop

Love-Lies-Bleeding ▲ — intense attachment to personal pain and suffering

Rock Rose ●✚ — shifting identification from body/ego to Higher Self

Sage ▲✚ — non-attachment to achievement or recognition

Sagebrush ▲✚ — to discern what is essential and let go of excess

Trillium ▲▼✚ — non-attachment to power and wealth

Nostalgia

Chrysanthemum ▲✚ — desire for youthfulness/attractiveness

Fairy Lantern ▲ — inability to accept maturity, longing to return to childhood

Forget-Me-Not ▲✚❖ — strong attachment to the memory of one who has died

Honeysuckle ●✚ — loneliness expressed as nostalgia

Nurturing (see Mothering)

Objectivity

Asclepias ▼ — objectivity in creative endeavors

Banana ■▲▼✚ — calmness, stepping back and observing, non-reactiveness

Carnation ✚ — emotional objectivity, the ability to meditate

Chrysanthemum ▲✚ — objective state to be more emotional/mental as required

Dill ▲▼♠ — objectivity and assimilation of incoming data

Garlic ▲✚ — cultivates objectivity rather than fear

Milkweed ▲✚ — mental clarity, objectivity, and spiritual consciousness

---

● BACH — ■ MASTER'S — ▲ FES — ▼ GREEN HOPE — ◆ AUSTRALIAN BUSH
❱ LIVING/AUSTRALIA — ❖ ALASKAN — ✚ PEGASUS — ✪ PERELANDRA

Queen Anne's Lace ▲▼✚ — objectivity in psychic awareness

Plum Tree ✚ — balanced and objective with spiritual and emotional realities

Purple and Red Kangaroo Paw ◗ — objective self analysis/rebalancing of partnerships

Purple Eremophila ◗ — serene objectivity amidst very personal issues of the heart

Radish ▼✚ — mental objectivity

Royal Ponciana ▼ — polite, detached, objective dialog no matter how sensitive topic

Sage ▲✚ — objectivity in looking at life experiences

Wooly Smokebush ◗ — perspective and humility

Obsession

Black Kangaroo Paw ◗ — grief/anger obsessive cycles

Blackberry ■▲▼✚ — obsessive thoughts and depression

Boronia ◆ — obsessive thoughts

Crab Apple ●▼✚ — obsessive concern with imperfection and impurities

Crown of Thorns ✚ — obsessions that lead to stress

Fig ■▲✚ — fanaticism

Filaree ▲✚ — obsessive concern over inessentials

Heather ●✚ — obsession with one's symptoms, compulsion to talk about problems

Horseradish ✚ — obsessive thought patterns discarded

Monkshood ▲✚✿ — obsession and extreme emotional imbalance

Orange (Citrus Aurantium) ✚ — subconscious emotional tensions, obsessive states

Orchid ✚ — cases of obsession, balances deep emotions

Pennyroyal ✚ — eases mental confusion and obsession

Pink Monkeyflower ▲ — obsessive-compulsive behaviors stemming from sex abuse

Purple Monkeyflower ▲ — obsessive-compulsive behaviors from ritual/occult abuse

Red Chestnut ●✚ — obsessive worry and concern about others

Rock Water ● — obsession with strict standards for oneself

Sticky Monkeyflower ▲ — obsessive/compulsive sexuality, fear of real intimacy

Vervain ●✚ — overzealous need to convert others
White Chestnut ● — obsessive thoughts

Optimism

Baby Blue Eyes ▲▼ — profound cynicism and paralysis of soul forces
Blackberry ■▲▼✚ — negativity, pessimism, sarcasm, cynicism
Borage ▲▼✚ — uplifts the heart, dispels gloom and sorrow, gives courage
Buttercup ▲✚ — a jaundiced view of life
California Wild Rose ▲✚ — cynical and apathetic attitude, no sense of destiny
Cape Bluebell ❱ — for issues of the past that leave a bitter taste
Cherry ■✚ — inspiration to others, optimistic, positive
Christ's Thorn ✚ — moving forward with optimism, peace and confidence
Dahlia ✚ — stimulates faith and confidence leading to optimism
Gentian ●✚ — giving up when difficulties are encountered
Golden Waitsia ❱ — to re-ignite spontaneity and carefree feelings
Gorse ●✚ — counteracting feelings of hopelessness, especially about personal affairs
Larch ●✚ — expecting failure, lack of belief in own talents/capacities
Oregon Grape ▲ — expecting hostility from others, "chip on shoulder"
Penstemon ▲✚ — perseverance despite hardships
Scotch Broom ▲✚ — seeing opportunity for service in spite of difficulties
Sunshine Wattle ◆ — acceptance of the beauty and joy in the present, optimism
Wallflower ✚ — stimulates joy and optimism
Wild Violet ❱ — fatalism and negativity about life in general
Yellow Flag Flower ❱ — keeping mind in positive frame

Organization (see Scattered)

Overview

Filaree ▲✚ — involvement with too many details
Quaking Grass ▲✚ — flexibility in group situations, seeing all sides
Rabbitbrush ▲✚ — mastery of many details

● BACH — ■ MASTER'S — ▲ FES — ▼ GREEN HOPE — ◆ AUSTRALIAN BUSH
❱ LIVING/AUSTRALIA — ❖ ALASKAN — ✚ PEGASUS — ✪ PERELANDRA

Sage ▲✚ — objectivity in looking at life experiences

Shasta Daisy ▲ — synthesis of many idea into one whole

Trillium ▲▼✚ — working for the greater whole

Overwhelm

Canyon Dudleya ▲ — overstimulated by life events

Chamomile ▲✚ — emotional hyperactivity

Cherry Plum ●✚ — fear that overwhelm will lead to breakdown/loss of control

Corn ■▲▼✚❂ — overwhelmed by city life

Cosmos ▲▼✚ — confusion from too many thoughts, especially when speaking

Dill ▲▼❂ — inundated by too many impressions and experiences

Elm ●✚ — responsibility too great, overextended and isolated

Hornbeam ● — intimidated by the tasks of everyday life

Indian Pink ▲✚ — overwhelmed by intensity of surrounding activity

Lavender ▲✚ — overwrought nerves

Oak ●✚ — going beyond natural limits

Pink Yarrow ▲ — taking on too much emotional intensity from others

Rabbitbrush ▲✚ — confusion from too many details

Red Clover ▲▼ — influenced by group emotions, hysteria, panic

Panic

Aspen ● — acute sensitivity to influences not seen or understood

Dog Rose of the Wild Forces ◆ — fear, loss of control, pain with no apparent cause

Emergency Care Solution ▼ — the Green Hope version of Rescue Remedy

Emergency Essence ◆ — the Australian Bush version of Rescue Remedy

Fuchsia Gum ◗ — panic in a confined space

Grey Spider Flower ◆ — terror, panic, nightmares from unknown causes

Kale ▲ — stress, fear, helplessness, panic

Many Headed Dryandra ◗ — panic/desire to run from responsibilities

Red Clover ▲▼ — influenced by group emotions, hysteria, panic

Rescue Remedy (Five Flower Formula) ● — to bring immediate calming

Rock Rose ●✚ — deep fear, terror, panic

● BACH — ■ MASTER'S — ▲ FES — ▼ GREEN HOPE — ◆ AUSTRALIAN BUSH
◗ LIVING/AUSTRALIA — ✤ ALASKAN — ✚ PEGASUS — ❂ PERELANDRA

St. John's Wort ▲▼✚ — panic disorder
Star of Bethlehem ●▼◗ — soothing/balancing in cases of shock, panic

Paranoia

Aspen ● — paranoia from fear of the unknown
Black Cohosh ▲ — suspicious of others, often from past violence/abuse
Garlic ▲✚ — eases fear and paranoia
Holly ●✚ — seeing others as unloving, unaccepting
Hybrid Pink Fairy/Cowslip Orchid ◗ — paranoia from psychic sensitivity
Kidney Bean ✚ — removes hidden anger, fear, paranoia
Oregon Grape ▲ — expecting hostility from others, paranoia
Pink Yarrow ▲ — absorbing emotions from others, uneasiness in
  crowds
Purple Monkeyflower ▲ — religious/spiritual beliefs leading to
  fear/paranoia
Pyrethrum ✚ — hidden fears, anxiety especially causing paranoia
Red Clover ▲▼ — hysteria/panic leading to paranoia
St. John's Wort ▲▼✚ — paranoia with sleep disorders
Spinach ■ — feeling burdened, overwhelmed with mild distrust to
  paranoia

Patience

Black-Eyed Susan ▲▼◆ — always on the go, impatience
Brown Boronia ◗ — patience and acceptance of the "here and now"
Buttercup ▲✚ — a jaundiced view of life
Coconut ■ — quitter, avoidance attitude
Cow Parsnip ✤ — eases impatience, dissatisfaction and anxiety during
  life changes
Crepe Myrtle ✚ — spiritual patience
Grape ■ — patience with others' shortcomings
Impatiens ●✚ — moderation of overly impulsive actions
Lettuce ■✚ — excitability, agitation
Lobelia ✚ — patience with self
Penstemon ▲✚ — perseverance and patience
Pine ● — increases tenacity and patience
Sycamore ✚ — strength, patience, constancy, endurance and persistence

---

● BACH — ■ MASTER'S — ▲ FES — ▼ GREEN HOPE — ◆ AUSTRALIAN BUSH
◗ LIVING/AUSTRALIA — ✤ ALASKAN — ✚ PEGASUS — ✪ PERELANDRA

Tomato ■▼✚✪ — knowing there is no failure

Yellow Leschenaultia ◗ — calms the mind

Perfectionism

Agrimony ●✚ — desire to appear emotionally perfect and acceptable, the "pleaser"

Alpine Lily ▲ — viewing female organs/sexuality as lower/imperfect

Beech ●✚ — blaming/criticizing others due to standards of perfectionism

Buttercup ▲✚ — inferiority complex, need to accept oneself

Centaury ● — slave to perfectionist standards of others

Cerato ●✚ — overdependence on others advice instead of learning from mistakes

Chamomile ▲✚ — difficulty dealing with challenging emotions of strife

Crab Apple ●▼✚ — obsessive concern with imperfection and impurities

Dandelion ▲▼✚✤ — over-planning life, enslaving body to impossible standards

Elm ●✚ — the hero, high standards of leading to frustration/overwhelm

Fawn Lily ▲ — secure in reclusive setting which is spiritually pure

Fig ■▲✚ — fanaticism

Filaree ▲✚ — obsession with petty worries

Gentian ●✚ — feeling lack of success means ultimate failure, inability to keep trying

Golden Waitsia ◗ — anxiety associated with perfectionism

Impatiens ●✚ — wanting everything to happen rapidly, easily irritated

Larch ●✚ — paralysis due to impossibility of achieving perfection, fear of mistakes

Lavender ▲✚ — high standards leading to oversensitivity, nervous affliction

Lobelia ✚ — courage to accept self as is, imperfections and all

Lotus ▲✚ — viewing self as spiritually advanced

Manzanita ▲✚ — seeing perfection only in what is spiritual

Pine ● — inability to forgive self, self-deprecation when less than perfect

Pretty Face ▲ — impossibly high standards of beauty

Red Chestnut ●✚ — over-concerned and overprotective

● BACH — ■ MASTER'S — ▲ FES — ▼ GREEN HOPE — ◆ AUSTRALIAN BUSH
◗ LIVING/AUSTRALIA — ✤ ALASKAN — ✚ PEGASUS — ✪ PERELANDRA

Rock Water ● — obsession with strict standards for oneself

Scarlet Monkeyflower ▲ — stuffing core anger and rage to appear nice

Vervain ●✚ — fanatical, overstriving

Vine ●✚ — expecting perfection from others

Water Violet ●✚ — drawing back from involvement with others, disdain for others

Willow ●✚ — resentment, blame of others

Yellow and Green Kangaroo Paw ❱ — for those frustrated by mistakes of others

Perseverance

Baby Blue Eyes ▲▼ — regaining trust and faith in spiritual destiny despite setbacks

Coconut ■ — quitter, avoidance attitude

Gentian ●✚ — perseverance despite setbacks, especially when discouraged or depressed

Kapok Bush ◆ — resignation, easily discouraged, apathy

Kolokoltchik ❱ — fought long/hard, cannot go on, accept defeat with head bowed

Larch ●✚ — continuing even after mistakes, learning from mistakes

Mountain Pride ▲✚ — warrior-like stamina in the face of adversity/challenge

Oak ●✚ — never-ceasing effort

Orange ■ — "might as well get used to it" attitude

Penstemon ▲✚ — perseverance and patience

Rosa Kamtchatica ✚ — ability to focus will and perseverance

Scotch Broom ▲✚ — overcoming negative or hopeless images of the world

Silver Princess Gum, Gungurra ❱ — perseverance when things don't work out

Washington Lily ✚ — spiritual perseverance

Wooly Banksia ❱ — desire to pursue ideals/goals when struggle seems too much

Personal Relationships

Almond ■▲✚ — addictive personality, sense of need

Basil ▲✚✺ — escaping commitment by deceptive/secret sexual behavior

● BACH — ■ MASTER'S — ▲ FES — ▼ GREEN HOPE — ◆ AUSTRALIAN BUSH
❱ LIVING/AUSTRALIA — ✣ ALASKAN — ✚ PEGASUS — ✺ PERELANDRA

Bleeding Heart ▲✚ — emotional freedom, ending co-dependent tendencies

Bush Gardenia ◆ — improves communication, passion

Buttercup ▲✚ — feeling worthless or low self-esteem

Calendula ▲▼✚ — listening to the other, non-interference and receptivity

California Wild Rose ▲✚ — listless and apathetic attitude

Chamomile ▲✚ — difficulty dealing with challenging emotions

Chicory ●✚ — emotional neediness

Crown of Thorns ✚ — holding back from life and relationship

Dogwood ▲ — grace and innocence in relationships

Evening Primrose ▲ — inability to form committed relationships

Fairy Lantern ▲ — immaturity, helplessness, neediness, childish dependency

Forget-Me-Not ▲✚❖ — understanding deeper meaning of relationships

Goldenrod ▲▼✚ — conforming to win approval

Grape ■ — patience with others' shortcomings

Heather ●✚ — obsession with one's symptoms, compulsion to talk about problems

Hibiscus ▲ — couples having difficulty relationship, like to discuss, fight all the time

Holly ●✚ — jealousy, envy

Ixora ▼ — sexual energy

Jojoba ✚ — helps participation in daily life and relationships

Lettuce ■✚ — indecisive, emotional congestion

Mallow ▲▼✚ — overcoming social barriers, developing trust and warmth

Mariposa Lily ▲ — receptivity to human love, nurturing

Mountain Wormwood ❖ — forgiveness of old wounds in relationships

Oregon Grape ▲ — expecting hostility from others, paranoia

Papaya ▲▼✚ — unity of mind, clarity of conscience in a relationship

Pear ■▲▼✚ — stability during major shifts/changes

Penstemon ▲✚ — perseverance and patience in relationships

Pine Drops ✚ — clear perspective on the entire nature of difficult relationships

Pink Monkeyflower ▲ — fear of intimacy/vulnerability, childhood shaming/abuse

Pink Yarrow ▲ — lack of emotional boundaries

● BACH — ■ MASTER'S — ▲ FES — ▼ GREEN HOPE — ◆ AUSTRALIAN BUSH
▶ LIVING/AUSTRALIA — ❖ ALASKAN — ✚ PEGASUS — ✪ PERELANDRA

Poison Oak ▲ — projecting hostility to keep others away

Purple Eremophila ◗ — serene objectivity amidst very personal issues of the heart

Quaking Grass ▲✚ — flexibility in group situations, seeing all sides

Rabbit Orchid ◗ — frustration with shallow, empty and obligatory relationships

Red Hibiscus ▼ — enhances compatibility between people in one-to-one relationship

Scarlet Monkeyflower ▲ — power and anger issues in relationships

Shooting Star ▲✚❖ — feeling at home, overcoming deep-seated alienation

Snapdragon ▲▼✚ — easily set off to make verbal attacks, snapping

Star Thistle ▲ — generosity and sharing in relationships

Sticky Monkeyflower ▲ — conflict/fear of intimacy in sexuality

Strawberry ■▲✚ — feeling unworthy, undeserving, irresponsible

Sunflower ▲▼✚❖ — healing father relationship, afflicted masculine aspect/animus

Sweet Pea ▲✚ — feeling cut off from community or family ties

Sweetgale ❖ — improving emotional communication in relationships

Tiger Lily ▲✚ — transmuting hostility and aggressiveness

Trillium ▲▼✚ — coveting the power/possessions of others, greed

Twinflower ❖ — balancing listening and speaking skills in relationships

Violet ▲ — shyness

Violet Butterfly ◗ — emotionally shattered during/after relationship traumas

Water Violet ●✚ — drawing back from involvement with others, disdain for others

Wedding Bush ◆ — difficulty with commitment in relationships

Yellow Star Tulip ▲ — sensitivity to the suffering of others

Perspective

Angel's Trumpet ▲✚ — viewing death as a transition rather than an ending

Angelica ▲▼✚ — awareness of benevolent spiritual forces

Banana ■▲▼✚ — calmness, stepping back and observing, non-reactiveness

Bloodroot ▲▼✚ — single point of focus, concentration, and meditation

Canyon Dudleya ▲ — shifting perspective to include ordinary events

---

● BACH — ■ MASTER'S — ▲ FES — ▼ GREEN HOPE — ◆ AUSTRALIAN BUSH
◗ LIVING/AUSTRALIA — ❖ ALASKAN — ✚ PEGASUS — ✪ PERELANDRA

Daffodil ▲▼✚ — deepens communication with entire self

Daisy ✚ — calm and centered amid intense activity, lightness, presence

Filaree ▲✚ — seeing petty concerns in the larger context

Forget-Me-Not ▲✚❖ — including spiritual world/beings in perception of daily life

Foxglove ▲❖✚ — seeing through limited perspective to the 'heart' of the matter

Fringed Lily Twiner ◗ — loss of balanced perspective leading to introversion

Green Rein Orchid ✚ — emotional perspective

Hound's Tongue ▲✚ — transforming overly materialistic perspective

Violet ▲ — spiritual perspective

Paper Birch ❖ — getting in touch with life purpose when faced with decisions

Pine Drops ✚ — clear perspective on the entire nature of difficult relationships

Queen Anne's Lace ▲▼✚ — objectivity in psychic awareness

Rabbitbrush ▲✚ — to see the big picture

Sage ▲✚ — objectivity in looking at life experiences

Scotch Broom ▲✚ — overcoming negative or hopeless images of the world

Shasta Daisy ▲ — synthesis of many idea into one whole

Silk Tree ✚ — promotes a transcendental perspective, inspiration, self-integration

Southern Cross ◆◗ — in touch with how life is experienced by others

Valerian ▲✚ — to gain perspective on priorities

White Eremophila ◗ — maintaining equipoise, consistency and direction in your life

White Spider Orchid ◗ — perspective on purpose of pain in journey of the soul

Wooly Smokebush ◗ — perspective and humility

Yellow Cone Flower ◗ — most important opinion is the one of yourself

Pessimism (see Optimism)

Possessiveness

Bleeding Heart ▲✚ — possessiveness in relationships from excessive dependence

Chicory ●✚ — emotional neediness
Grape ■ — loving without condition, demand or expectation
Star Thistle ▲ — stinginess, inability to share self or possessions
Trillium ▲▼✚ — coveting the power/possessions of others, greed

Power

Black Cohosh ▲ — transforming darker psychic energy, wrestling inner demons
Blackberry ■▲▼✚ — lack of strong forces of will
California Pitcher Plant ▲✚ — weakness or excess strength of instinctual forces
Centaury ● — controlled by others' expectations, resisting exploitative relationships
Chicory ●✚ — being manipulative in relationships especially from insecurity/neediness
Chrysanthemum ▲✚ — attachment to power and position, fear of death
Fairy Lantern ▲ — giving away personal power, feigning helplessness
Horseradish ✚ — strength and empowerment
Lady's Slipper ▲✤ — spiritual forces not fully grounded and integrated
Larkspur ▲✚ — providing leadership with joy, charisma
Mountain Pride ▲✚ — warrior-like stamina in the face of adversity/challenge
Nicotiana ▲ — appearing powerful/in control by numbing/suppressing feelings
Pale Sundew ◗ — rapacious, manipulative power playing
Pineapple ■✚ — confidence, empowerment
Pink Yarrow ▲ — giving personal power away by "bleeding" into others' energy
Quince ▲✚ — conflicts between power and love in feminine forces
Quinoa ✚ — grounding, gets people beyond power trips
Rosa Castilian ✚ — greater sense of inner energy, compassion in the use of power
Scarlet Monkeyflower ▲ — power and anger issues in relationships
Shy Blue Orchid ◗ — dynamism where powerlessness previously prevailed
Sitka Spruce Pollen ✤ — balancing power and gentleness in men and women

Snapdragon ▲▼✚ — strong vital power/magnetism turning to verbal abuse

Soapberry ✿ — balancing one's personal power with the power of nature

Southern Cross ◆❱ — personal power, positive attitude, taking responsibility

Spinifex ◆❱ — empowerment through emotional understanding

Sunflower ▲▼✚✿ — balanced power and ego strength, radiant individuality

Tiger Lily ▲✚ — transmuting hostility and aggressiveness

Trillium ▲▼✚ — coveting the power/possessions of others, greed

Vine ●✚ — domination of others

Pregnancy

Alpine Lily ▲ — experiencing reproductive organs in positive way

Angelica ▲▼✚ — spiritual protection for the incoming child

Bleeding Heart ▲✚ — letting go of a miscarried or aborted child

Borage ▲▼✚ — sooth heart pain after miscarriage/abortion

California Wild Rose ▲✚ — for difficult pregnancies

Calla Lily ▲✚ — mixed messages about sexual identity in utero

Cerato ●✚ — developing trust in inner knowing

Chamomile ▲✚ — balancing emotional ups and downs

Cherry Plum ●✚ — extremely stressful pregnancy or labor

Corn ■▲▼✚✪ — grounding and centering in the body

Easter Lily ▲✚ — cleansing of sexual organs, especially when conception is blocked

Evening Primrose ▲ — destructive intent to the fetus during pregnancy

Forget-Me-Not ▲✚✿ — contacting the incarnating spirit

Gorse ●✚ — postpartum depression

Hybrid Pink Fairy/Cowslip Orchid ❱ — sensitivity of pregnancy

Lady's Mantle ✚ — for fertility, pregnancy and birth

Lavender ▲✚ — nervous stress and oversensitivity

Manzanita ▲✚ — acceptance of physical body during pregnancy

Mugwort ▲✚ — overdue pregnancy

Mullein ▲✚ — deciding whether to carry a child

Olive ●✚ — fatigue from missed sleep, exhaustion from long labor

Penstemon ▲✚ — perseverance in difficult pregnancy

Pink Yarrow ▲ — oversensitivity to emotions of others

Pomegranate ▲▼✚ — conflict between family and career

Quince ▲✚ — conflicts between power and love in feminine forces

Red Chestnut ●✚ — worry and concern about pregnancy/new child

Scleranthus ●✚ — doubts/indecision about life changes from pregnancy

Shooting Star ▲✚✤ — for possible miscarriage, premature birth, difficult labor

Star Tulip ▲✚ — developing receptivity as a mother

Walnut ●✚ — transition on each stage of pregnancy, releasing child at birth

Yarrow ▲ — vulnerability to negative influences

Yarrow Special Formula ▲ — protection from environmental pollution/disharmony

Yellow Star Tulip ▲ — telepathic communication with child

Watermelon ▲✚ — to eliminate emotional stress during pregnancy

Zucchini ▲▼✚✪ — harmonious pregnancy

Prejudice

Angelica ▲▼✚ — to see the spiritual core rather than outer physical characteristics

Beech ●✚ — negative image of others, critical

Black-Eyed Susan ▲▼◆ — seeing others as bad/evil due to repression of psyche

Boab ◆ — release of abusive thought patterns from family

Buttercup ▲✚ — internalizing stereotypes projected from others

Calendula ▲▼✚ — inability to listen to what others are really saying

Canyon Dudleya ▲ — inciting mass hysteria or derogatory stereotypes

Centaury ● — internalizing master-slave relationship

Date ■ — closed, intolerant, irritable

Deerbrush ▲ — out of touch with real feelings

Fig ■▲✚ — fanaticism

Goldenrod ▲▼✚ — conforming to win approval

Holly ●✚ — indicated for prejudice of any kind, inclusive, not exclusive

Honeysuckle ●✚ — inability to accept current social reality

Mountain Pride ▲✚ — taking a stand for truth or social justice

Mullein ▲✚ — developing a sense of conscience

● BACH — ■ MASTER'S — ▲ FES — ▼ GREEN HOPE — ◆ AUSTRALIAN BUSH
◗ LIVING/AUSTRALIA — ✤ ALASKAN — ✚ PEGASUS — ✪ PERELANDRA

Oregon Grape ▲ — seeing other groups as violent/undesirable

Penstemon ▲✚ — perseverance despite prejudice

Pine ● — self-blame, feeling one is bad or unworthy

Pretty Face ▲ — inability to see racial characteristics as beautiful

Quaking Grass ▲✚ — for groups, communities to work in harmony

Red Clover ▲▼ — hysteria/panic leading to paranoia

Saguaro ▲✚ — overcoming prejudicial beliefs or superstitions

Slender Rice Flower ◆ — racism formed from personal experience, narrow minded

Vervain ●✚ — fanatical belief in ideology or political program

Vine ●✚ — domination of others

Walnut ●✚ — breaking old ties that are prejudicial

Water Violet ●✚ — feeling superior by virtue of culture, class or race

Pride

Banana ■▲▼✚ — false pride

Buttercup ▲✚ — healthy pride in accomplishments

Gymea Lily ◆ — arrogant, attention seeking, craving status/glamour, dominating

Larch ●✚ — pride and confidence in creativity, especially when doubting abilities

Lotus ▲✚ — spiritual pride

Magnolia ▲✚ — pride and dignity

Pineapple ■✚ — confidence, empowerment

Pretty Face ▲ — healthy pride in appearance, inner beauty illuminates physical

Slender Rice Flower ◆ — humility

Strawberry ■▲✚ — quiet sense of self and self-worth

Sunflower ▲▼✚✣ — egotistical sense of self-importance, overbearing individuality

Water Violet ●✚ — excessive pride, aloofness, feeling better than others

Procrastination

Blackberry ■▲▼✚ — putting ideas into action, overcoming inertia

Cayenne ▲✚ — cutting through stagnation or indecision

Clematis ●✚ — avoidance of tasks at hand, dreamy disposition

Coconut ■ — quitter, avoidance attitude

● BACH — ■ MASTER'S — ▲ FES — ▼ GREEN HOPE — ◆ AUSTRALIAN BUSH
◗ LIVING/AUSTRALIA — ✣ ALASKAN — ✚ PEGASUS — ✪ PERELANDRA

Corn ■▲▼✚✪ — sluggishness, dragging one's feet, lethargy

Cosmos ▲▼✚ — for introverted, shy, procrastinating people

Hornbeam ● — lack of energy due to emotional resistance to work

Jacaranda ◆ — scattered, changeable, dithering, unfocused, rushing

Larch ●✚ — putting off action out of fear of failure, lack of confidence

Pumpkin ▼✚ — procrastination

Sundew ◆ — daydreaming, procrastinating, disconnected, spaced out, lack of focus

Tansy ▲✚ — procrastinating, lethargic, overly phlegmatic, indecisive

Protection

Angel of Protection ✚ — vulnerability, need of protection

Angelica ▲▼✚ — protection/nurturing from spiritual guides

Angelsword ◆ — spiritual protection

Fringed Violet ◆ — psychic protection

Garlic ▲✚ — protection from psychic parasites which drain vitality

Golden Yarrow ▲ — protection despite innate sensitivity

Lavender ▲✚ — soothing when exposed to too much nervous stimulation

Mariposa Lily ▲ — protection of child from harmful influences

Monkshood ▲✚✤ — creating a sacred space for deep inner work

Mountain Pennyroyal ▲ — expelling negative psychic forces

Pennyroyal ✚ — protection from others' negative thoughts

Pink Yarrow ▲ — emotional vulnerability

Poison Oak ▲ — overly defensive and self-protective

Purple Monkeyflower ▲ — feeling protection, trust regarding spiritual experience

Red Clover ▲▼ — insulation from hysteria/panic

St. John's Wort ▲▼✚ — protection during dreaming, trust in divine protection

Shy Blue Orchid ◗ — protection/dynamism where powerlessness used to prevail

Tomato ■▼✚✪ — psychic protection

Walnut ●✚ — freedom from outside ideas and influences that stymie or subvert

White Violet ✤ — protection from having functional energetic boundaries

---

Yarrow ▲ — protection from negative thoughts or influences

Yarrow Special Formula ▲ — protection from noxious influences in environment

Yellow Yarrow ▲▼✪ — emotional protection during vulnerable times

Psychic Abilities (see Clairvoyance)

Psychosomatic Illness

Arnica ▲✚ — releasing past trauma which mask insight into current illness

Canyon Dudleya ▲ — conditions come and go rapidly, appear worse than are

Fawn Lily ▲ — weakness, fatigue, fragile or delicate temperament

Fuchsia ▲ — emotional repression manifesting as acute illness, headaches

Lavender ▲✚ — headaches/nervous problems from overstimulation of spirit

Pink Monkeyflower ▲ — sexual/bodily dysfunction from soul shame/violation

Pomegranate ▲▼✚ — PMS, etc. from unresolved feelings of creativity/reproduction

Queen Anne's Lace ▲▼✚ — distortions in vision, masking emergent clairvoyance

Scleranthus ●✚ — shifting symptoms, constant energetic changes

Self-Heal ▲ — contacting true source of healing, self-responsibility

Star of Bethlehem ●▼❱ — soothing/reorienting body to soul-spiritual self

Wild Rose ● — sickness that lingers, loss of interest in life

Yerba Santa ▲✚ — tendency toward respiratory illness from melancholia

Purification

Blackberry ■▲▼✚ — sloughing off the old

Chaparral ▲✚ — cleansing of subconscious emotions/psychic toxins

Crab Apple ●▼✚ — over-concern with physical toxins

Deerbrush ▲ — clarity in the heart to inner intentions, especially with mixed motives

Easter Lily ▲✚ — purification of emotions centered in sexual organs

---

● BACH — ■ MASTER'S — ▲ FES — ▼ GREEN HOPE — ◆ AUSTRALIAN BUSH
❱ LIVING/AUSTRALIA — ❖ ALASKAN — ✚ PEGASUS — ✪ PERELANDRA

Evening Primrose ▲ — cleansing toxic psychic emotions absorbed in utero/infancy

Fireweed ▲✢✚ — regeneration, purification

Golden Ear Drops ▲ — toxic childhood memories in heart, deep crying

Grass of Parnassus ✢ — purification of immediate environment

Lotus ▲✚ — purifies emotions

Mountain Pennyroyal ▲ — cleansing psychic infestation

Noni ▲ — cleanses emotions to prepare women for childbearing and motherhood

Plantain ▲ — mental cleansing and purification

Sagebrush ▲✚ — shedding false identity, releasing what is no longer essential

Star Tulip ▲✚ — spiritual purification

Sweetgrass ✢ — purification of etheric body

Quiet

Aconite ✚ — deep inner quiet

Almond ■▲✚ — calmness of the mind

Angelica ▲▼✚ — protection/nurturing from spiritual guides

Bachelor's Button ✚ — sense of gentleness/quiet with ability to express ideas

Banana ■▲▼✚ — calmness, stepping back and observing, non-reactiveness

Chamomile ▲✚ — emotional quietude and calm

Indian Pink ▲✚ — inner stillness despite intense activity

Lettuce ■✚ — "the unruffler"

Madia ▲✚ — inner silence and concentration

Peony ▲✚ — quiets the mind

Sage ▲✚ — inner peace and equanimity, especially from life experience/reflection

Sagebrush ▲✚ — deep emptiness, pregnant silence as way of stilling soul

Solomon's Seal ✚ — brings quietness and detachment

Star Tulip ▲✚ — inner peace and receptivity, inner listening

Strawberry ■▲✚ — quiet sense of self and self-worth

Valerian ▲✚ — quiet, restful, help for insomnia

White Chestnut ● — mental repose

Rebelliousness

Almond ■▲✚ — immoderation

Jasmine ▲▼✚ — rebelliousness

Red Helmet Orchid ◆ — rebellious, problems with authority

Red Beak Orchid ❭ — adolescence/mid-life frustrations with duties and family ties

Saguaro ▲✚ — delinquent/destructive behavior from rebellion against authority

Silver Princess Gum, Gungurra ❭ — to care, not give up or rebel

Receptivity

Angelica ▲▼✚ — receptivity to guidance/guardianship from angelic realms

Calendula ▲▼✚ — hearing the message and intent of another

Chiming Bells ✤ — receptivity of the angelic kingdom

Coffee ▲✚ — receptivity to vibrational medicines

Date ■ — contentment with receptivity, open-mindedness, magnetic nature

Forget-Me-Not ▲✚✤ — openness to spiritual guides/karmic connections

Hollyhock ▲✚ — feminine softness, receptivity, open and compassionate heart

Icelandic Poppy ✤ — receptivity to spiritual power

Jacob's Ladder ✤✚ — receiving creative impulses of the soul

Lamb's Quarters ✤ — mental receptivity by opening channel between heart/mind

Lotus ▲✚ — openness to higher spiritual awareness

Mallow ▲▼✚ — receiving the warmth and love of others

Mariposa Lily ▲ — receptivity to human love, mother-child bonding

Mugwort ▲✚ — keeping psychic balance as intuitive faculties are opening

Mullein ▲✚ — hearing the voice of conscience

Sagebrush ▲✚ — emptiness as a precondition to change and transformation

Star Tulip ▲✚ — receptivity to spiritual worlds, listening to inner voice

Sweetgale ✤ — emotional receptivity

Violet ▲ — openness to warmth of others in a group

White Violet ✤ — creating function boundaries to support receptivity

Yellow Star Tulip ▲ — emotional receptivity, empathy

Rejection

Angelica ▲▼✚ — taken care of by higher forces despite rejection by others

Baby Blue Eyes ▲▼ — early rejection/lack of support becoming cynicism/mistrust

Black Cohosh ▲ — addiction to relationships despite rejection or abuse

Bleeding Heart ▲✚ — feeling spurned by lover/partner, emotional attachment

Buttercup ▲✚ — feeling insignificant compared to others

Chicory ●✚ — overly needy, never enough love or support

Crab Apple ●▼✚ — feeling dirty, unclean, not good enough, not pure enough

Dogwood ▲ — awkward, accident-prone, feeling unlovable, a victim

Echinacea ▲✚ — devastated and shattered by abuse/trauma, loss of essential dignity

Evening Primrose ▲ — rejection/abandonment in utero/infancy, fear of rejection

Gentian ●✚ — discouragement due to rejection/failure

Goldenrod ▲▼✚ — fear of social censure

Holly ●✚ — feeling unloved, jealous, envious

Holly Thorn ✚ — fear of rejection

Honeysuckle ●✚ — dealing with rejection by dwelling on past

Illawara Flame Tree ◆ — sense of rejection, being left out

Larch ●✚ — expecting rejection or failure

Mallow ▲▼✚ — difficulty initiating/sustaining friendships

Mariposa Lily ▲ — estrangement from mother leading to feelings of rejection

Oregon Grape ▲ — projection/expectation of hostility leading to rejection

Pine ● — self-blame, feeling one is bad or unworthy

Pink Monkeyflower ▲ — profound shame

Pretty Face ▲ — feeling ugly

Scarlet Monkeyflower ▲ — believes will be rejected if strong emotions are expressed

Shooting Star ▲✚❖ — feeling rejected by human community

Sticky Monkeyflower ▲ — fear of intimacy and rejection

Sweet Chestnut ●✚ — feeling abandoned by God, hopeless and alone

---

● BACH — ■ MASTER'S — ▲ FES — ▼ GREEN HOPE — ◆ AUSTRALIAN BUSH
◗ LIVING/AUSTRALIA — ❖ ALASKAN — ✚ PEGASUS — ✪ PERELANDRA

Sweet Pea ▲✚ — feeling cut off from community or family ties

Willow ●✚ — dwells on feelings of rejection leading to bitterness

Rejuvenation

Almond ■▲✚ — synchronicity of body/mind/spirit

Aloe Vera ▲▼✚ — reviving exhausted creative forces

Baby Blue Eyes ▲▼ — restoration of childlike innocence and trust in soul

California Wild Rose ▲✚ — awakening to life, enthusiasm, involvement

Coriander ✚ — hatred rejuvenated into passion

Date Palm ▼✚ — rejuvenates DNA

Hibiscus ▲ — rejuvenation when sexuality is depleted

Indian Paintbrush ▲✚ — to revive creative expression

Iris ▲ — re-awakening of artistic abilities, especially higher inspiration

Loofa (Lufa) ▲✚ — rejuvenates the body

Morning Glory ▲▼✚ — fresh "morning" forces depleted by erratic sleep/drugs

Nasturtium ▲▼✚❍ — awaken body when depleted from too much intellectual work

Olive ●✚ — re-invigoration after long struggle or physical exhaustion

Rosa Gallica Officinalis ✚ — spiritual rejuvenation

Self-Heal ▲ — contacting true source of healing

Sweetgrass ❖ — rejuvenation of etheric body

Relationship (see Personal Relationship)

Relaxation

Balm-Lemon ✚ — calms

Bougainvillaea ▼✚ — relaxes body

Canyon Dudleya ▲ — to calm overexcited or hysterical tendencies

Chamomile ▲✚ — emotional quietude and calm

Comfrey ▲▼✚❍ — releases nervous tension and improves memory

Dampiera ❱ — letting go and letting life flow

Dandelion ▲▼✚❖ — release of tension and stress held in body

Dill ▲▼❍ — difficulty relaxing from overstimulation

Elm ●✚ — letting go of undue worry

Emergency Care Solution ▼ — the Green Hope version of Rescue Remedy

Emergency Essence ◆ — the Australian Bush version of Rescue Remedy

Fig ■▲✚ — at ease with self and others, relaxation

Hops Bush ◗ — can't sleep or relax from frenetic energy

Kangaroo Paw ◆ — relaxed, sensitivity, savior faire, enjoyment of people

Lavender ▲✚ — overwrought nerves

Lettuce ■✚ — "the unruffler"

Lilac ▲▼✚ — mental clarity and relaxation

Magnolia ▲✚ — increases sense of freedom and relaxation

Milk Thistle ✚ — relaxes and dissolves emotions

Mock Orange ✚ — stress reduction

Monterey Pine ✚ — deep relaxation

Morning Glory ▲▼✚ — nervousness due to erratic life patterns/addictions

Purple Flag Flower ◗ — releasing pressure and tension

Ragweed-Ambrosia ✚ — relaxes emotions

Red Chestnut ●✚ — tension due to excessive anxiety and worry about others

Rescue Remedy (Five Flower Formula) ● — to bring immediate calming

Rose Campion ✚ — relaxing, balancing

Tiare ✚ — deep relaxation

Valerian ▲✚ — promotes relaxation, contentment

Vervain ●✚ — moderation, de-stressing

White Chestnut ● — letting go of obsessive, repetitive thoughts directed inward

Release

Alpine Azalea ❖ — release of self-doubt

Amaranthus ✚ — releases stress

Angel's Trumpet ▲✚ — letting go of physical body in dying process

Artichoke ✚ — release grief and sadness

Balsam Poplar ❖ — releasing sexual tension stemming from abuse

Bittersweet ✚ — releases grief, mourning and despondency

Bleeding Heart ▲✚ — releasing unhealthy attachments

Blue Elf Viola ❖ — release of anger and frustration

● BACH — ■ MASTER'S — ▲ FES — ▼ GREEN HOPE — ◆ AUSTRALIAN BUSH
◗ LIVING/AUSTRALIA — ❖ ALASKAN — ✚ PEGASUS — ❍ PERELANDRA

Blueberry Pollen ❖ — releasing mental limitations

Boab ◆ — release of abusive thought patterns from family

Breadfruit ✚ — releases tension related specifically to sexual dysfunction

Bunchberry ❖ — releasing attachment to distraction

Catnip ✚ — releases stress and irrational fear

Chamomile ▲✚ — releasing nervousness and emotional tension

Cherry Plum ●✚ — overcoming fear of losing control

Chestnut Bud ●✚ — releasing old habit patterns

Chicory ●✚ — to let go of emotional neediness/need for attention

Chives ▼✪ — releases power and energy

Chrysanthemum ▲✚ — acceptance of mortality

Cotton Grass ❖ — letting go of pain held in the body

Cucumber ▼✪ — release of fear

Daffodil ▲▼✚ — releases frustration of self-criticism

Dampiera ❱ — letting go and letting life flow

Dandelion ▲▼✚❖ — release of tension and stress held in body

Desert Barrel Cactus ✚ — releasing boundaries

Dogwood ▲ — release of hardened emotions from past trauma

Evening Primrose ▲ — releasing toxic emotions absorbed in infancy

Filaree ▲✚ — letting go of trivial/petty worries

Forget-Me-Not ▲✚❖ — releasing pain held deep in subconscious

Forsythia ▲ — releasing outdated patterns of behavior

Foxglove ▲❖✚ — releasing emotional tension around heart

Fuchsia ▲ — releasing false or hyper-emotionality

Ginseng ✚ — clarity and release of creativity

Golden Ear Drops ▲ — releasing childhood emotional pain, especially by crying

Graniana Rose ▼ — breaking up blockages to creative expression

Green Bog Orchid ❖ — sensitivity through release of pain/fear held deep in heart

Green Spider Orchid ◆ — release of terrors, nightmares, phobias

Hollyhock ▲✚ — releasing negativity

Honeysuckle ●✚ — releasing nostalgia

Hyssop ▲▼✚ — releases tension throughout body

Jacob's Ladder ❖✚ — releasing need to mentally control events of our lives

---

● BACH — ■ MASTER'S — ▲ FES — ▼ GREEN HOPE — ◆ AUSTRALIAN BUSH
❱ LIVING/AUSTRALIA — ❖ ALASKAN — ✚ PEGASUS — ✪ PERELANDRA

Laceflower ❖ — release of negative or false self-image

Ladies' Tresses ❖ — for releasing deeply held traumas

Love-Lies-Bleeding ▲ — understand/release intense pain/suffering

Macrozamia ◗ — release blockages brought about by sexual trauma

Mahogany ✚ — grounding, release negative thoughts

Marjoram ✚ — emotional release, especially fear

Mountain Pennyroyal ▲ — expulsion of negative thoughts, especially those from others

Mountain Wormwood ❖ — releasing resentment toward self or others

Oak ●✚ — knowing when to let go of struggle

Onion ▲✚ — release of birth trauma

Orange (Citrus Aurantium) ✚ — Releases emotional tensions stored in subconscious

Passion Flower ▲▼✚ — release of tension

Peony ▲✚ — releases creative blocks and fear of intimacy

Pink Monkeyflower ▲ — release of emotional fears and shame, especially rejection

Plantain ▲ — release rigid or negative thought patterns that keep us stuck

Potato ✚ — cleanse and release what we no longer need to carry around

Purple Flag Flower ◗ — releasing pressure and tension

Raspberry ■✚ — "turning the other cheek," releasing old wounds, forgiveness

Rose Campion ✚ — releases hurt

Sagebrush ▲✚ — to shed false identity

Sassafras ✚ — releases stress

Soapberry ❖ — release of fear of power and nature

Sphagnum Moss ❖ — releasing judgement form the heart

Sticky Geranium ❖ — releasing inner potential

Sweetgale ❖ — release of emotional tension in relationships

White Chestnut ● — letting go of obsessive, repetitive thoughts directed inward

White Fireweed ❖ — releasing emotional shock

Yerba Santa ▲✚ — release of past emotional trauma stored in psyche

Zucchini ▲▼✚◒ — releases creativity

● BACH — ■ MASTER'S — ▲ FES — ▼ GREEN HOPE — ◆ AUSTRALIAN BUSH
◗ LIVING/AUSTRALIA — ❖ ALASKAN — ✚ PEGASUS — ◒ PERELANDRA

Repression

Agrimony ●✚ — repressing real feelings due to politeness/superficial standards

Black-Eyed Susan ▲▼◆ — lack of awareness of one's shadow side

Bluebell ◆ — cut off from feelings

Centaury ● — repressing need for expression in order to please others

Chaparral ▲✚ — cleansing of subconscious emotions/psychic toxins

Dandelion ▲▼✚✣ — holding tense emotions in the body

Everlasting ✚ — repressed childhood memories

Evening Primrose ▲ — repression of core emotions and sexual feelings

Fuchsia ▲ — repression of true emotions, often covered by false emotionality

Golden Ear Drops ▲ — repression of painful childhood memories

Hibiscus ▲ — inhibition of sexuality

Larch ●✚ — blockage of creative expression

Lettuce ■✚ — emotional repression

Nicotiana ▲ — repression of feeling life in the heart, especially with addiction

Pink Monkeyflower ▲ — holding back true feelings of intimacy/love from shame

Purple Monkeyflower ▲ — unconscious fear of the occult

Red Hibiscus ▼ — repression of sexual trauma

Rock Water ● — self-repression through over-strictness

Scarlet Monkeyflower ▲ — holding back/denying anger/strong emotions from fear

Snapdragon ▲▼✚ — repressed metabolic and libido energy, with anger

Sticky Monkeyflower ▲ — inhibition of sexual feelings due to fear of intimacy

Tansy ▲✚ — suppression of energy/feelings to keep peace

Vine ●✚ — trying to repress free will of others

Yerba Santa ▲✚ — constriction of emotions, especially sadness/grief

Resentment

Baby Blue Eyes ▲▼ — cynical/detached preventing feeling goodness of others

Black Kangaroo Paw ◗ — resentment of parents, other authority figures growing up

---

● BACH — ■ MASTER'S — ▲ FES — ▼ GREEN HOPE — ◆ AUSTRALIAN BUSH
◗ LIVING/AUSTRALIA — ✣ ALASKAN — ✚ PEGASUS — ✪ PERELANDRA

Dagger Hakea ◆ — resentment, bitterness toward family

Holly ●✚ — jealousy, envy

Milk Thistle ✚ — resentment or other held feelings which block the flow of love

Mountain Wormwood ❖ — releasing resentment toward self or others

Oregon Grape ▲ — resentment, seeing other people's actions in negative light

Raspberry ■✚ — blame, resentment, bitterness

Watermelon ▲✚ — resentment, "so mad you can't speak," anger

Willow ●✚ — blaming others, bitterness

Resignation

California Wild Rose ▲✚ — resigned and apathetic

Gorse ●✚ — despair, hopelessness about personal affairs

Kapok Bush ◆ — resignation, easily discouraged, apathy

Orange ■ — "might as well get used to it" attitude

Plantain ▲ — turning resignation into acceptance

Star of Bethlehem ●▼◗ — feeling there is no way out

Wild Rose ● — apathy/resignation when faced with illness/challenge

Resilience

Dandelion ▲▼✚❖ — resilience of body

Orange ■ — cultivating an inner smile

Willow ●✚ — resilience of mind

Resistance

Agrimony ●✚ — denial of emotional pain as a way to resist doing inner work

Angel's Trumpet ▲✚ — fear of death, resistance to letting go of life

Bauhinia ◆ — resistance to change

Black-Eyed Susan ▲▼◆ — difficulty penetrating into shadow aspects of personality

Blackberry ■▲▼✚ — overcoming resistance to manifestation

Bog Rosemary ❖ — overcoming resistance to being healed

California Wild Rose ▲✚ — resisting pain by disengaging from life

Cayenne ▲✚ — breaking through resistance, catalyzing will

Cerato ●✚ — resisting inner guidance

● BACH — ■ MASTER'S — ▲ FES — ▼ GREEN HOPE — ◆ AUSTRALIAN BUSH
◗ LIVING/AUSTRALIA — ❖ ALASKAN — ✚ PEGASUS — ✪ PERELANDRA

Chestnut Bud ●✚ — not learning lessons of experience

Chrysanthemum ▲✚ — difficulty accepting aging process

Clematis ●✚ — resistance to being in present by daydreaming/fantasizing

Corn ■▲▼✚✪ — sluggishness, dragging one's feet, resistance

Dandelion ▲▼✚✤ — emotional holding expressed as muscular tension

Fairy Lantern ▲ — resisting adult responsibilities

Fuchsia ▲ — resistance to true feelings, often expressed as false emotionality

Golden Ear Drops ▲ — difficulty contacting childhood emotions

Harebell ✤ — resistance to receiving love from universal sources

Honeysuckle ●✚ — resistance to being in the present

Hornbeam ● — lack of energy due to emotional resistance to work

Impatiens ●✚ — not accepting the seemingly slow pace of life/others

Manzanita ▲✚ — resistance to healing due to aversion to physical incarnation

Morning Glory ▲▼✚ — difficulty facing day due to depletion of vitality

Pink Monkeyflower ▲ — holding back true feelings of intimacy/love from shame

Poison Oak ▲ — resisting social/intimate contact, fear of having boundaries violated

Quaking Grass ▲✚ — difficulty working with group process

Rock Water ● — rigidity, inflexibility, difficulty opening up to feelings

Saguaro ▲✚ — resistance to authority

Scarlet Monkeyflower ▲ — holding back/denying anger/strong emotions from fear

Self-Heal ▲ — inner resistance to taking responsibility for own healing process

Spiraea ✤ — resistance to growth and expansion

Star Thistle ▲ — resistance to sharing with others

Star Tulip ▲✚ — resistance to inner work, spiritual receptivity

Tansy ▲✚ — resistance to true expression of one's energy

Water Violet ●✚ — aversion to social involvement

Willow ●✚ — overcoming mental resistance

Responsibility

Alpine Mint Bush ◆ — weight of responsibility

● BACH — ■ MASTER'S — ▲ FES — ▼ GREEN HOPE — ◆ AUSTRALIAN BUSH
◗ LIVING/AUSTRALIA — ✤ ALASKAN — ✚ PEGASUS — ✪ PERELANDRA

Blue Topped Cow Weed ◗ — sense of responsibility
Centaury ● — feeling overly responsible for others
Chicory ●✚ — feeling responsible for others in a possessive, clinging way
Christmas Tree (Kanya) ◗ — to fulfill family responsibilities
Elm ●✚ — overburdened/overwhelmed by responsibility
Fairy Lantern ▲ — resisting adult responsibilities
Illawara Flame Tree ◆ — fear of responsibility
Larkspur ▲✚ — providing leadership with joy, charisma
Many Headed Dryandra ◗ — panic/desire to run from responsibilities
Mountain Pride ▲✚ — social responsibility
Oak ●✚ — easily accepting responsibility due to strong abilities
Peach Flowered Tea Tree ◆ — taking responsibility for own health
Raspberry ■✚ — taking responsibility for actions
Red Beak Orchid ◗ — conflict between desires/duties, expression/responsibilities
Red Chestnut ●✚ — feeling responsible for the problems of others
Red Feather Flower ◗ — sharing burdens in family/community life
Southern Cross ◆◗ — personal power, positive attitude, taking responsibility
Strawberry ■▲✚ — feeling unworthy, undeserving, irresponsible
Sweet Pea ▲✚ — sense of social responsibility
Willow ●✚ — taking responsibility for life rather than blaming others
Wintergreen ▼✚ — cleanses sense of false responsibility

Restlessness

Almond ■▲✚ — calmness of the mind
California Poppy ▲▼ — constant fascination with psychic techniques/religious cults
Canyon Dudleya ▲ — dissatisfaction with quiet/ordinary pace of life
Dill ▲▼✪ — difficulty relaxing from overstimulation
Impatiens ●✚ — restlessness due to impatient, quick temperament
Lady's Slipper ▲✿ — restlessness with nervous exhaustion and sexual depletion
Lavender ▲✚ — nervous and sensitive, tendency toward insomnia, high strung
Lettuce ■✚ — "the unruffler"

Licorice ✚ — calms restlessness

Magnolia ▲✚ — eases restlessness and lack of clarity

Morning Glory ▲▼✚ — nervous problems from erratic lifestyle, chaotic habits

Red Beak Orchid ◗ — conflict between desires/duties, expression/responsibilities

Scleranthus ●✚ — indecisiveness, constant alternation between choices

W.A. Smokebrush ◗ — difficult concentration, vagueness, feeling muddled

White Chestnut ● — mental restlessness, constant chatter of thought

Wild Oat ● — trying many vocations but unable to find life purpose

Rigidity

Bauhinia ◆ — resistance to change

Beech ●✚ — hard, judgemental, demanding, unrealistic perfectionism

California Bay Laurel ✚ — rigid mindset

Dampiera ◗ — rigidity of mind and body

Dandelion ▲▼✚✤ — rigid thinking

Fig ■▲✚ — fanaticism

Goldenrod ▲▼✚ — rigid religious beliefs

Hibbertia ◆ — rigid personality, fanaticism about self-improvement

Lilac ▲▼✚ — rigidity in the body

Plantain ▲ — release rigid or negative thought patterns that keep us stuck

Rock Water ● — rigidity, inflexibility, difficulty opening up to feelings

Spruce ▲✚ — accepting one's own fallibility, willingness to compromise

Water Violet ●✚ — keeping one's distance from others, disdain, elitism, racism

Sadness (see Depression)

Sarcasm

Blackberry ■▲▼✚ — negativity, pessimism, sarcasm, cynicism

Snapdragon ▲▼✚ — verbal abuse/biting sarcasm

Scatteredness

Clematis ●✚ — resistance to being in present by daydreaming/fantasizing

● BACH — ■ MASTER'S — ▲ FES — ▼ GREEN HOPE — ◆ AUSTRALIAN BUSH
◗ LIVING/AUSTRALIA — ✤ ALASKAN — ✚ PEGASUS — ✪ PERELANDRA

Daisy ✚ — calm and centered amid intense activity, lightness, presence

Emergency Care Solution ▼ — the Green Hope version of Rescue Remedy

Emergency Essence ◆ — the Australian Bush version of Rescue Remedy

Hops Bush ◗ — excessive and scattered energy

Indian Pink ▲✚ — overwhelmed by intensity of surrounding activity

Jacaranda ◆ — scattered, changeable, dithering, unfocused, rushing

Lettuce ■✚ — indecisive, emotional congestion, too many thoughts at once

Madia ▲✚ — short attention span, flits from one activity to another

Pomegranate ▲▼✚ — scattered energy

Rabbitbrush ▲✚ — confusion from too many details

Rescue Remedy (Five Flower Formula) ● — to bring immediate calming

Scleranthus ●✚ — indecisiveness, constant alternation between choices

Shasta Daisy ▲ — scattered thinking

Sweet Pea ▲✚ — for the constant wanderer or traveler unable to establish roots

Wild Oat ● — trying many vocations but unable to find life purpose

Searching/Seeking

California Poppy ▲▼ — constant fascination with psychic techniques/religious cults

Cerato ●✚ — seeking the advice of others, overly dependent on outside validation

Daisy ✚ — stabilizes those who are constantly seeking but not finding

Goldenrod ▲▼✚ — desiring others' approval, negative attention for disapproval

Rabbit Orchid ◗ — for those who want to find their true and deeper self

Self-Heal ▲ — seeking various healing forms without inner willingness to be healed

Sweet Alyssum ✚ — seeking to transcend dogmatic religious states

Sweet Pea ▲✚ — lack of connectedness and roots, the perpetual seeker

Wild Oat ● — trying many vocations but unable to find life purpose

Yucca ✚ — seek the truth beyond the appearance or "looks-as-if"

Self-Acceptance/Self-Appreciation

Alpine Azalea ✤ — release of self-doubt

Alpine Lily ▲ — acceptance of female self

● BACH — ■ MASTER'S — ▲ FES — ▼ GREEN HOPE — ◆ AUSTRALIAN BUSH
◗ LIVING/AUSTRALIA — ✤ ALASKAN — ✚ PEGASUS — ✪ PERELANDRA

Baby Blue Eyes ▲▼ — feeling at ease with self, letting down guard

Billy Goat Plum ◆ — self-disgust and dislike of the body, especially the sex organs

Bird of Paradise ✚ — viewing self as unsightly or ugly

Buttercup ▲✚ — accepting the worth of one's life, vocation or lifestyle

Columbine ❖ — building a strong projection of one's identity

Crab Apple ●▼✚ — acceptance of self instead of focus on impurities/imperfections

Echinacea ▲✚ — reclaiming positive spiritual identity

Fig ■▲✚ — at ease with self

Five Corners ◆ — love and acceptance of self, celebration of own beauty

Lace Flower ❖ — appreciation of one's contributions to humanity

Larch ●✚ — confidence in inner strength and abilities

Mariposa Lily ▲ — warm and loving acceptance of self

Milkmaids ✚ — sweetness, love and acceptance of self

Penstemon ▲✚ — accepting handicaps or afflictions

Pine ● — self-blame, feeling one is bad or unworthy

Pineapple ■✚ — judging self in comparison to others

Pretty Face ▲ — feeling ugly

Self-Heal ▲ — contacting true source of healing

Sunflower ▲▼✚❖ — ability to shine, emanate true self, believe in self

Tiger Lily ▲✚ — self-appreciation and self-acceptance

Self-Actualization

Baby Blue Eyes ▲▼ — moving forward despite harsh experience

Blackberry ■▲▼✚ — putting ideas into action, overcoming inertia

Buttercup ▲✚ — accepting the worth of one's life, vocation or lifestyle

Centaury ● — developing strong sense of self

Chrysanthemum ▲✚ — shift from ego-identification to higher spiritual identity

Cosmos ▲▼✚ — capacity for higher thought, integration of mental/spiritual

Echinacea ▲✚ — sense of wholeness, despite threats to inner self

Gladiola ✚ — increase in sensitivity, ability to assimilate information, awareness

Golden Yarrow ▲ — feeling protected despite innate sensitivity

---

● BACH — ■ MASTER'S — ▲ FES — ▼ GREEN HOPE — ◆ AUSTRALIAN BUSH
❱ LIVING/AUSTRALIA — ❖ ALASKAN — ✚ PEGASUS — ✪ PERELANDRA

Iris ▲ — awakening of artistic abilities, especially higher inspiration

Lady's Slipper ▲❖ — to ground and integrate spiritual forces

Milkweed ▲✚ — estrangement from core self, can't cope with normal demands

Mullein ▲✚ — fulfillment of true potential

Quince ▲✚ — conflict between showing strength and emotional warmth

Self-Heal ▲ — taking responsibility for own well-being, facing karma

Sunflower ▲▼✚❖ — ability to shine, emanate true self, believe in self

Tansy ▲✚ — procrastinating, lethargic, overly phlegmatic, indecisive

Wild Oat ● — finding the inner calling to a vocation

Self-Concern

Chicory ●✚ — overly needy, never enough love or support

Crab Apple ●▼✚ — feeling dirty, unclean, not good enough, not pure enough

Fawn Lily ▲ — overemphasis on spiritual activity, insulating self from the world

Filaree ▲✚ — letting go of trivial/petty worries

Heather ●✚ — obsession with one's symptoms, compulsion to talk about problems

Love-Lies-Bleeding ▲ — understand/release intense pain/suffering

Mimulus ●✚ — nervousness from everyday fears and worries

Self-Discipline

Almond ■▲✚ — immoderation

Hibbertia ◆ — rigid personality, fanaticism about self-improvement

Blue China Orchid ◗ — to strengthen will and take back control of self

Chickweed ✚ — in need of self-discipline

Fig ■▲✚ — fanaticism

Green Rose ✚◗ — maintaining disciplines and healthy habits

Jacob's Ladder ❖✚ — releasing need to mentally control events of our lives

Onion ▲✚ — lack of discipline, illogical, irrational

Rice ✚ — habits related to discipline needs like smoking, sadomasochism

Rock Water ● — rigidity, inflexibility, difficulty opening up to feelings

Silver Princess Gum, Gungurra ◗ — perseverance when things don't work out

Sycamore ✚ — strength, patience, constancy, endurance and persistence

Self-Effacement

Billy Goat Plum ◆ — self-disgust and dislike of the body, especially the sex organs

Bird of Paradise ✚ — viewing self as unsightly or ugly

Buttercup ▲✚ — belittling self

Centaury ● — being a doormat for others

Fairy Lantern ▲ — feigning helplessness/dependency, playing the child

Larch ●✚ — expecting failure, lack of belief in own talents/capacities

Mimulus ●✚ — fretful and fearful, seeing self as weak and vulnerable

Pine ● — self-blame, feeling one is bad or unworthy

Pink Monkeyflower ▲ — emotional masking, shame

Pretty Face ▲ — feeling ugly

Sunflower ▲▼✚❖ — suppression of individuality, lack of strong sense of self

Violet ▲ — shyness

Self-Esteem

Apple ■▲✚ — hope, motivation, a positive outlook

Billy Goat Plum ◆ — self-disgust and dislike of the body, especially the sex organs

Bird of Paradise ✚ — viewing self as unsightly or ugly

Black-Eyed Susan ▲▼◆ — emotional honesty to examine shadow side of self

Brazil Nut ✚ — develops self-esteem and more confidence in decision making

Buttercup ▲✚ — knowing true worth

Calla Lily ▲✚ — ability to integrate sexual identity with sense of self

Centaury ● — serving others out of self- worth, not servitude

Cerato ●✚ — strength to follow inner guidance

Columbine ❖ — building a strong projection of one's identity

Correa ◗ — from inner acceptance—to focus—to success

Cosmos ▲▼✚ — capacity for higher thought, integration of mental/spiritual

---

● BACH — ■ MASTER'S — ▲ FES — ▼ GREEN HOPE — ◆ AUSTRALIAN BUSH
◗ LIVING/AUSTRALIA — ❖ ALASKAN — ✚ PEGASUS — ✪ PERELANDRA

Daffodil ▲▼✚ — replaces depression/low self-worth with love and trust

Echinacea ▲✚ — sense of wholeness

Evening Primrose ▲ — rejection/abandonment in utero/infancy, fear of rejection

Fairy Lantern ▲ — inability to see self as full-fledged adult

Five Corners ◆ — love and acceptance of self, celebration of own beauty

Ginseng ✚ — improves self esteem

Goldenrod ▲▼✚ — individuality and strength

Heather ●✚ — seeing self in terms of one's problems

Jasmine ▲▼✚ — purifies the ego, cleanses the individual of negative self images

Larch ●✚ — expecting failure, lack of belief in own talents/capacities

Lion's Tail ✚ — develops self-esteem

Lotus ▲✚ — seeing self as expression of spirituality

Mallow ▲▼✚ — confidence in social situations

Milkmaids ✚ — sweetness, love and acceptance of self

Persimmon ▲✚ — low self-esteem, sexual inhibitions, lack of proper sexual identity

Pretty Face ▲ — feeling ugly

Purple Monkeyflower ▲ — can't contact core spiritual identity from ritual abuse

Sage ▲✚ — ability to view self within larger panorama of events

Sagebrush ▲✚ — shedding false identity, releasing what is no longer essential

Snakebush ◗ — fulfilling self-love

Solomon's Seal ✚ — emotional instability, low self-esteem, and over-inquisitiveness

Strawberry ■▲✚ — feeling unworthy, undeserving, irresponsible

Sturt Desert Rose ◆ — to follow inner convictions and morality

Sunflower ▲▼✚✣ — ability to shine, emanate true self, believe in self

Tamarack ✣ — awareness of true essence, self-confidence/understanding abilities

Trumpet Vine ▲✚ — healthy self-assertion, especially speaking up/asserting self

Urchin Dryandra ◗ — self worth, understanding of how one got into victimhood

Wakiki Rainbow Cactus ✚ — self worth, positive self expression
Yellow Cone Flower ◗ — most important opinion is the one of yourself

Self-Expression

Beech ●✚ — tendency to make critical comments

Buttercup ▲✚ — increased sense of inner confidence and self-worth when speaking

Calendula ▲▼✚ — expressing warmth, intimacy and nurturing feelings with words

Cosmos ▲▼✚ — nervous speech patterns which are too rapid

Heather ●✚ — seeking social contact by talking excessively about problems

Iris ▲ — artistic impulses in speaking, poetry and drama

Larch ●✚ — confidence in expression

Mountain Pride ▲✚ — courage to take risks, to stand up and speak out

Raspberry ■✚ — taking responsibility for actions

Snapdragon ▲▼✚ — verbal abuse/biting sarcasm

Sunflower ▲▼✚✤ — boastful, drawing attention to self and accomplishments

Trumpet Vine ▲✚ — healthy self-assertion, especially speaking up/asserting self

Violet ▲ — shyness

Wakiki Rainbow Cactus ✚ — self worth, positive self expression

Selfishness

Bleeding Heart ▲✚ — emotional attachments, co-dependent relationships

Blue Leschenaultia ◗ — rekindles the desire to give with grace and benevolence

Chicory ●✚ — overly needy, never enough love or support

Chrysanthemum ▲✚ — accumulating wealth/power to make life permanent

Fawn Lily ▲ — spiritual selfishness

Fringed Lily Twiner ◗ — demanding, overconcentration on self

Heart Orchid ✚ — transmuting selfish emotions into love

Heather ●✚ — obsession with one's symptoms, compulsion to talk about problems

Holly ●✚ — inability to feel love or admiration for others

● BACH — ■ MASTER'S — ▲ FES — ▼ GREEN HOPE — ◆ AUSTRALIAN BUSH
◗ LIVING/AUSTRALIA — ✤ ALASKAN — ✚ PEGASUS — ✪ PERELANDRA

Peach ■▲✚ — selfishness, self-involvement, "looking out for Number One"

Red Helmet Orchid ◆ — rebelliousness, selfish, problems with authority

Solomon's Seal ✚ — egoism, selfishness, superiority, obnoxious

Star Thistle ▲ — stinginess, feeling of lack, not sharing

Trillium ▲▼✚ — seeking personal gain and power

Water Violet ●✚ — keeping one's distance from others, disdain, elitism

Yellow Star Tulip ▲ — lack of awareness of what others are feeling

Sensitivity

Angelica ▲▼✚ — feeling protected and guided

Aspen ● — hypersensitive to things unseen or unknown

Beech ●✚ — oversensitive leading to hypercritical nature

Calendula ▲▼✚ — hearing the message and intent of another

Chamomile ▲✚ — subject to emotional tension

Chaparral ▲✚ — absorbing disturbing or violent images

Date ■ — sensitive to others

Golden Yarrow ▲ — feeling protected despite innate sensitivity

Hybrid Pink Fairy/Cowslip Orchid ❱ — psychic sensitivity

Jojoba ✚ — for those unable to cope with the mundane

Lavender ▲✚ — nervous and sensitive, tendency toward insomnia, high strung

Love-Lies-Bleeding ▲ — intense attachment to personal pain and suffering

Mezereon ✚ — increases sensitivity

Mountain Pennyroyal ▲ — negative thoughts/thinking patterns taken on from others

Mugwort ▲✚ — awareness of dreams, conscious control of psychic life

Nicotiana ▲ — inability to cope with sensitivity, numb/deaden soul experiences

Northern Twayblade ❖ — grounding sensitivity into physical experience

Orange Leschenaultia ❱ — brings in touch with softness of life, empathy reemerges

Pink Fairy Orchid ❱ — stress from environmental chaos or pressure

Pink Monkeyflower ▲ — extreme sensitivity with emotional masking, shame

Pink Yarrow ▲ — absorbing emotions from others

Poison Oak ▲ — projecting hostility to keep others away

Purple Eremophila ◗ — serene objectivity amidst very personal issues of the heart

Purple Monkeyflower ▲ — extreme fear or apprehension from spiritual/occult

Queen Anne's Lace ▲▼✚ — to integrate emotions, sexuality with psychic life

Red and Green Kangaroo Paw ◗ — in touch with loved ones, promoting sensitivity

Red Chestnut ●✚ — obsessive worry and concern about others

Red Grevillia ◆ — feeling stuck, affected by criticism, reliant on others

Red Leschenaultia ◗ — essence of gentleness and sensitivity

Ruta (Rue) ▲✚ — extreme vulnerability to others and to the environment

St. John's Wort ▲▼✚ — overexpanded psyche

Sensitive Plant ✚ — extremely shy and withdrawn or introverted

Star of Bethlehem ●▼◗ — soothing acute sensitivity and trauma

Star Tulip ▲✚ — receptivity to spiritual worlds

Walnut ●✚ — freedom from outside ideas and influences that stymie or subvert

White Violet ✤ — energetic support for those highly sensitive

Yarrow ▲ — protection from negative thoughts or influences

Yarrow Special Formula ▲ — protection from noxious influences in environment

Yellow Star Tulip ▲ — emotional receptivity, empathy

Zucchini ▲▼✚✪ — increases sensitivity in men

Seriousness

Canyon Dudleya ▲ — allowing small episodes to appear overly dramatic

Fairy Lantern ▲ — to develop more depth and seriousness

Fig ■▲✚ — rigidity, tension, uncompromising nature

Hornbeam ● — approaching life as a dull routine, lack of joy

Little Flannel Flower ◆ — denial of "child" in self, too serious

Nasturtium ▲▼✚✪ — over intellectualization, lacking vitality

Rock Water ● — rigidity, inflexibility, difficulty opening up to feelings

Spinach ■ — feeling burdened, overwhelmed

Vervain ●✚ — fanatical belief in ideology or political program

---

● BACH — ■ MASTER'S — ▲ FES — ▼ GREEN HOPE — ◆ AUSTRALIAN BUSH
◗ LIVING/AUSTRALIA — ✤ ALASKAN — ✚ PEGASUS — ✪ PERELANDRA

Wild Oat ● — becoming more serious/directed about life and vocation

Zinnia ▲▼✚✪ — taking money/business too seriously, need to enjoy life

Service

Centaury ● — serving others out of self-worth, not servitude

Fawn Lily ▲ — protecting and nurturing others

Larkspur ▲✚ — providing leadership with joy, charisma

Leafless Orchid ◗ — feelings of depletion for those who work in service to others

Lime ▼✚ — transmuting self-preservation into detached world service

Mariposa Lily ▲ — developing mothering forces, serving children

Money Plant ✚ — attitude of service and understanding of its real meaning

Mountain Pride ▲✚ — courage to take risks, to stand up and speak out

Purple Nymph Waterlily ◗ — selfless service

Scotch Broom ▲✚ — seeing world difficulties as opportunities for service

Tiger Lily ▲✚ — sense of receptivity and cooperation

Trillium ▲▼✚ — working for the greater whole

Vine ●✚ — transforming tyrannical tendencies to positive service for others

Water Violet ●✚ — sharing, overcoming aloofness or pride

White Spider Orchid ◗ — brings love and caring to darkest corners of the world

Yellow Star Tulip ▲ — emotional receptivity, empathy

Sexuality

Aggression Orchid ✚ — aggressive, impulsive, sexual aggression

Almond ■▲✚ — wholesome sexuality

Alpine Lily ▲ — viewing female organs/sexuality as lower/imperfect

Balga (Blackboy) ◗ — maturing of the male principle within

Balsam Poplar ✣ — releasing sexual tension stemming from abuse

Banana ■▲▼✚ — balances male sexuality

Banksia Baxtena ✚ — balance in male sexuality

Banksia Marginata ✚ — balances male psychological problems concerning sexuality

---

● BACH — ■ MASTER'S — ▲ FES — ▼ GREEN HOPE — ◆ AUSTRALIAN BUSH
◗ LIVING/AUSTRALIA — ✣ ALASKAN — ✚ PEGASUS — ✪ PERELANDRA

Basil ▲✚✪ — secrecy and deception in sexual behavior

Billy Goat Plum ◆ — self-disgust and dislike of the body, especially the sex organs

Black Cohosh ▲ — abusive, exploitative, incestuous relationships

Breadfruit ✚ — releases tension related specifically to sexual dysfunction

California Pitcher Plant ▲✚ — fear of the instinctual aspects of the self

Calla Lily ▲✚ — uncertainty and confusion about sexual identity

Castor Bean ✚ — balanced sexual identity

Coconut ■ — hidden fears or emotional imbalances, especially concerning male sexuality

Crab Apple ●▼✚ — feeling of shame, that sexuality is unclean

Dogwood ▲ — hardening of sexual forces, especially from trauma or abuse

Easter Lily ▲✚ — alternating between promiscuity and prudishness

Evening Primrose ▲ — repression of core emotions and sexual feelings

Fairy Lantern ▲ — tendency to stay in prepubescent sexuality

Flannel Flower ◆ — uncomfortable with physical/emotional intimacy

Fuchsia ▲ — sexual feelings sublimated into psychosomatic emotions

Ginseng ✚ — sexual anxiety

Goddess Grasstree ◗ — maturing of the female principle from within

Grape ■ — healthy sexuality

Hibiscus ▲ — inhibition of sexuality

Ixora ▼ — sexual energy, relationship-enhancer for heterosexual couples

Lady's Slipper ▲✤ — depletion of sexual forces with nervous exhaustion

Larch ●✚ — men: can't measure up, feeling inadequate

Lobelia ✚ — express, own and speak the truth of one's sexuality

Macadamia ✚ — inhibited sexuality

Macrozamia ◗ — release blockages brought about by sexual trauma

Manzanita ▲✚ — accepting the body, feeling good about physical nature

Mariposa Lily ▲ — healing sexual abuse from childhood

Onion ▲✚ — domestic violence/sexual abuse

Orange ■ — physical, emotional or sexual abuse

Papaya ▲▼✚ — helps resolve identity crises connected with one's sexuality

Persimmon ▲✚ — aphrodisiac, sexual inhibitions, lack of sexual sensitivity

---

● BACH — ■ MASTER'S — ▲ FES — ▼ GREEN HOPE — ◆ AUSTRALIAN BUSH
◗ LIVING/AUSTRALIA — ✤ ALASKAN — ✚ PEGASUS — ✪ PERELANDRA

Pink Monkeyflower ▲ — shame of sexual organs from past abuse

Pistachio ✚ — desire to curb sexual appetite, promiscuity, desire for monogamy

Poinsettia ✚ — oversexed or sexually repressed

Pomegranate ▲▼✚ — conflicts about feminine procreative instinct

Purple Monkeyflower ▲ — ritual sexual abuse involving cultish beliefs

Queen Anne's Lace ▲▼✚ — to integrate emotions, sexuality with psychic life

Red Ginger ✚ — male/female union, sexuality

Red Hibiscus ▼ — repression of sexual trauma

Red Leschenaultia ◗ — harshness/brittle attitudes stopping love/joy/closeness

Snapdragon ▲▼✚ — repressed metabolic and libido energy, with anger

Sticky Monkeyflower ▲ — inhibition of sexual feelings due to fear of intimacy

Wisteria ◆ — fulfillment and enjoyment of sexuality

Ylang Ylang ✚ — sexual stress

Yucca ✚ — suppressed sexual energy

Zucchini ▲▼✚✪ — creativity, balance, strength, clarifying regarding sexuality

Shadow Consciousness

Baby Blue Eyes ▲▼ — cynical/detached preventing feeling goodness of others

Black Cohosh ▲ — transforming darker psychic energy, wrestling inner demons

Black-Eyed Susan ▲▼◆ — emotional honesty to examine shadow side of self

California Pitcher Plant ▲✚ — fear of the instinctual aspects of the self

Illyarrie ◗ — to deal with past shadows and pain

Scarlet Monkeyflower ▲ — holding back/denying anger/strong emotions from fear

Snapdragon ▲▼✚ — repressed metabolic and libido energy, with anger

Vine ●✚ — darkened forces of the will which control others

Shame

Agrimony ●✚ — covering shame with a mask of cheerfulness

Alpine Lily ▲ — shame based on distorted image of female sexuality

Basil ▲✚✪ — shame-producing or aberrant sexual behavior

Bougainvillaea ▼✚ — releases guilt, shame

Buttercup ▲✚ — sense of worthlessness, feeling unimportant

Calla Lily ▲✚ — shame/confusion about sexual orientation

Crab Apple ●▼✚ — feeling of shame, that one is unclean, impure

Easter Lily ▲✚ — feeling sexuality is impure, unspiritual, lower

Golden Ear Drops ▲ — repressed childhood memories of shame

Larch ●✚ — fear of being shamed

Lobelia ✚ — shame and fear of one's sexual nature

Pine ● — self-blame, feeling one is bad or unworthy

Pink Monkeyflower ▲ — profound shame

Poison Ivy ▲✚ — to go from feeling shamed to feeling blessed

Pretty Face ▲ — feeling ugly

Purple Monkeyflower ▲ — shame stemming from occult or ritual abuse

Scarlet Monkeyflower ▲ — feels emotional shadow is shameful, dangerous

Sharing

Bluebell ◆ — opens the heart, joy, sharing

Calendula ▲▼✚ — communicating warmly with others

Centaury ● — knowing limits in sharing, ability to say no

Chicory ●✚ — giving love without the need to get something in return

Christmas Tree (Kanya) ◗ — to fulfill family and group responsibilities

Fawn Lily ▲ — sharing spiritual gifts with others

Grape ■ — loving without condition, demand or expectation

Holly ●✚ — opening heart to receive and give love

Mallow ▲▼✚ — developing friendship and social warmth

Monkshood ▲✚❖ — sharing physical space through spiritual agreement

Pink Monkeyflower ▲ — opening up to others despite fear

Purple Nymph Waterlily ◗ — selfless service

Red Feather Flower ◗ — sharing burdens in family/community life

Star Thistle ▲ — giving of oneself to others

Trillium ▲▼✚ — working for the greater whole

Violet ▲ — sense of individuality when sharing with a group

Water Violet ●✚ — sharing, overcoming aloofness or pride

Wild Iris ❖ — sharing inner beauty and creative energy

● BACH — ■ MASTER'S — ▲ FES — ▼ GREEN HOPE — ◆ AUSTRALIAN BUSH
◗ LIVING/AUSTRALIA — ❖ ALASKAN — ✚ PEGASUS — ✪ PERELANDRA

Shattered Feelings

Cowkicks ❱ — despair after physical trauma

Echinacea ▲✚ — devastated and shattered by abuse/trauma, loss of essential dignity

Sagebrush ▲✚ — deep emptiness

Violet Butterfly ❱ — emotionally shattered during/after relationship traumas

Waratah ◆ — black despair, hopelessness, inability to respond to crisis

Shock

Arnica ▲✚ — healing past shock or trauma

Cotton Grass ❖ — recovering from shock to physical body

Echinacea ▲✚ — devastated and shattered by abuse/trauma

Emergency Care Solution ▼ — the Green Hope version of Rescue Remedy

Emergency Essence ◆ — the Australian Bush version of Rescue Remedy

Fireweed ▲❖✚ — recovering from shock to physical body

Horseradish ✚ — in shock: creates mental clarity

Horsetail ❖✚ — for slight shock or trauma

Ladies' Tresses ❖ — for releasing deeply held traumas

Lavender ▲✚ — shock to the nerves from too many spiritual forces in body

Pear ■▲▼✚ — for any troubling experience: accidents, shock, etc.

Pink Monkeyflower ▲ — violation/abuse leading to emotional closing/shame

Radish ▼✚ — integrates mind after shock, trauma, bereavement

Rescue Remedy (Five Flower Formula) ● — overall recovery from shock/trauma

River Beauty ❖ — emotional re-orientation and recovery after shock

Rosa Damascena Bifera (Damask Rose) ✚ — sudden mental shock

St. John's Wort ▲▼✚ — nervous depletion from out-of-body experiences

Scarlet Runner Bean ▼ — trauma/shock

Self-Heal ▲ — recuperative healing from shock

Star of Bethlehem ●▼❱ — soothing acute sensitivity and trauma

Sweetgrass ❖ — rejuvenation of etheric body

White Fireweed ❖ — releasing emotional shock

● BACH — ■ MASTER'S — ▲ FES — ▼ GREEN HOPE — ◆ AUSTRALIAN BUSH
❱ LIVING/AUSTRALIA — ❖ ALASKAN — ✚ PEGASUS — ❂ PERELANDRA

Shyness

Banana ■▲▼✚ — anxiety, nervousness

Bluebell ◆ — opens the heart, joy, sharing

Buttercup ▲✚ — lack of self-worth, of having something of value to share

Dog Rose ◆ — fearful, shy, apprehensive of others, niggling fears

Golden Glory Grevillea ◗ — for those who withdraw rather than deal with criticism

Happy Wanderer ◗ — trepidation

Hybrid Pink Fairy/Cowslip Orchid ◗ — extra-sensitive to others' judgements

Larch ●✚ — expecting failure, lack of belief in own talents/capacities

Mallow ▲▼✚ — difficulty initiating/sustaining friendships

Mimulus ●✚ — fretful and fearful, seeing self as weak and vulnerable

Pineapple ■✚ — inferiority complex

Sensitive Plant ✚ — extremely shy and withdrawn or introverted, eases stress

Strawberry ■▲✚ — feeling unworthy, undeserving

Tomato ■▼✚✪ — fear, withdrawal

Violet ▲ — fear of losing oneself in a group

Water Violet ●✚ — keeping one's distance from others, aloofness

Sleep (see Insomnia, Dreams)

Sluggish

Blackberry ■▲▼✚ — putting ideas into action, overcoming inertia

Cayenne ▲✚ — breaking through resistance, catalyzing will

Corn ■▲▼✚✪ — sluggishness, dragging one's feet, resistance

Cosmos ▲▼✚ — for introverted, shy, procrastinating people

Hornbeam ● — intimidated by the tasks of everyday life

Horseradish ✚ — boredom, lethargy, depression, or hysteria

Morning Glory ▲▼✚ — difficulty facing day due to depletion of vitality

Old Man Banksia ◆ — disheartened, weary, phlegmatic

Peppermint ▲✚ — lightness in thinking, mental alertness

Red Beak Orchid ◗ — renews energy and inspiration

Robinia ✚ — for the overly lethargic individual

Rubber Tree ✚ — for lack of concentration, lethargy, and spaciness

Sugar Cane ✚ — sharp mood swings, lethargy, and general depression

Sycamore ✚ — strength, patience, constancy, endurance and persistence

Tansy ▲✚ — procrastinating, lethargic, overly phlegmatic, indecisive

Tea Plant ✚ — overcoming mental lethargy, stagnation

Softness

Baby Blue Eyes ▲▼ — restoration of childlike innocence and trust

Calendula ▲▼✚ — expressing warmth, intimacy and nurturing feelings with words

Deerbrush ▲ — purity of feelings within the heart

Dogwood ▲ — release of hardened emotions from past trauma

Golden Yarrow ▲ — remaining in contact with others, softening without merging

Hollyhock ▲✚ — feminine softness, receptivity, open and compassionate heart

Jacaranda ◆ — softness and grace

Mariposa Lily ▲ — developing mothering forces

Motherwort ✚ — inner softness, outer strength

Orange Leschenaultia ❱ — brings in touch with softness of life, empathy reemerges

Pine ● — increases tenacity and patience

Pink Monkeyflower ▲ — showing softer, more vulnerable emotions

Poison Ivy ▲✚ — to go from feeling shamed to feeling blessed

Poison Oak ▲ — fear of soft/feminine side, projecting hostility to keep others away

Quince ▲✚ — conflict between showing strength and emotional warmth

Sycamore ✚ — restores gentleness and smoothness to energy flow

Yellow Star Tulip ▲ — emotional receptivity, empathy

Soothing

Calendula ▲▼✚ — expressing warmth, intimacy and nurturing feelings with words

Chamomile ▲✚ — releasing nervousness and emotional tension

Comfrey ▲▼✚✪ — releases nervous tension and improves memory

Lavender ▲✚ — soothes overwrought nerves

Lettuce ■✚ — "the unruffler"

● BACH — ■ MASTER'S — ▲ FES — ▼ GREEN HOPE — ◆ AUSTRALIAN BUSH
❱ LIVING/AUSTRALIA — ✤ ALASKAN — ✚ PEGASUS — ✪ PERELANDRA

Mariposa Lily ▲ — mothering forces of protection and comfort
Marjoram ✚ — emotional release, especially fear
Purple Nightshade ✚ — soothes jangled, burned-out nervous states
Star of Bethlehem ●▼❱ — soothing acute sensitivity and trauma

Soulfulness

Alpine Lily ▲ — greater inner space for the feminine self
Angelica ▲▼✚ — perceiving/receiving help from higher worlds
Deerbrush ▲ — purity of feelings within the heart
Forget-Me-Not ▲✚❖ — awareness of spiritual/karmic factors in relationships
Holly ●✚ — ability to feel soul connection with others
Iris ▲ — creating inner vessel for receiving higher inspiration
Sagebrush ▲✚ — experiencing inner space within the soul
Star Tulip ▲✚ — receptivity to spiritual worlds
Yellow Star Tulip ▲ — emotional receptivity, empathy
Yerba Santa ▲✚ — restoring sanctity of the heart center

Speaking

Brussel Sprouts ✚ — trouble speaking before the public
Calendula ▲▼✚ — contacting healing power of the word
Canyon Dudleya ▲ — to calm and harmonize speech which excites others
Cinnamon ✚ — for a clearer expression of one's feelings
Cosmos ▲▼✚ — nervous speech patterns which are too rapid
Garlic ▲✚ — fear when speaking, stage fright
Golden Yarrow ▲ — projecting voice despite anxiety
Heather ●✚ — compulsion to talk about problems
Hybrid Pink Fairy/Cowslip Orchid ❱ — nervous speaking in public
Larch ●✚ — confidence in self-expression
Leopard Lily ✚ — to express self more clearly
Lettuce ■✚ — ability to speak one's truth
Madia ▲✚ — scattered, unfocused talking
Mimulus ●✚ — shyness, timidity, swallowing words, nervousness when speaking
Red Clover ▲▼ — speech full of fear and anxiety absorbed from others
Rosa Virginia ✚ — inner sense of calmness and stillness in words

---

● BACH — ■ MASTER'S — ▲ FES — ▼ GREEN HOPE — ◆ AUSTRALIAN BUSH
❱ LIVING/AUSTRALIA — ❖ ALASKAN — ✚ PEGASUS — ✪ PERELANDRA

Snapdragon ▲▼✚ — lashing out, using cutting or biting words

Sunflower ▲▼✚❖ — projecting positive self-image when speaking

Trumpet Vine ▲✚ — healthy self-assertion, especially speaking up/asserting self

Twinflower ❖ — balancing listening and speaking skills in relationships

Vervain ●✚ — intense beliefs imposed on others

White Chestnut ● — repetitive chattering

Spiritual Emergency or Opening

Angel's Trumpet ▲✚ — experiencing death as genuine spiritual experience

Angelica ▲▼✚ — protection when opening to spiritual experience

Angelsword ◆ — spiritual protection

Arnica ▲✚ — soul remains connected to physical body after trauma

Aspen ● — fear of the unknown when crossing a spiritual threshold

Baby Blue Eyes ▲▼ — soul feels estranged from spiritual world

Banksia Baxtena ✚ — spiritual impotency

Bougainvillaea ▼✚ — reaffirm commitment to spiritual destiny

Bush Iris ◆ — spiritual insight

California Poppy ▲▼ — fascination or glamour in spiritual experiences

Canyon Dudleya ▲ — unbalanced/hysterical states of psychism/mediumism

Cherry-Sweet ✚ — spiritual identity

Chin Cactus ✚ — spiritual loneliness

Corn ■▲▼✚✪ — grounding spiritual energy through the body

Crepe Myrtle ✚ — spiritual patience

Desert Barrel Cactus ✚ — sadness felt in spiritual journey

Fawn Lily ▲ — craving spiritual/meditation experience as a retreat from life

Forget-Me-Not ▲✚❖ — connection with spiritual guides

Garlic ▲✚ — drained due to fear of the spiritual world

Ginseng ✚ — spiritual awareness

Golden Corydalis ❖ — spiritual focus for the development of the personality

Green Rose ✚◗ — spiritual healing

Icelandic Poppy ❖ — receptivity to spiritual power

Indian Paintbrush ▲✚ — polarizing currents between heaven and earth

Iris ▲ — bringing more soulful aspects to spiritual identity

Lady's Slipper ▲❖ — integration of inner spiritual authority with real life tasks

Lavender ▲✚ — harsh/strenuous spiritual practices leading to nervous overload

Lilac ▲▼✚ — facilitates the flow of spiritual energy

Lotus ▲✚ — seeing self as expression of spirituality

Love-Lies-Bleeding ▲ — seeing larger spiritual purpose/meaning when suffering

Mahogany ✚ — psycho-spiritual disorientation

Mandrake ✚ — ego death and spiritual rebirth

Mango ✚ — spiritual growth and alignment

Milkweed ▲✚ — over-dependence on spiritual leaders or dogma

Money Plant ✚ — balance between material and spiritual desires

Mountain Pennyroyal ▲ — invaded or taken over by other entities

Mugwort ▲✚ — awareness of dreams, conscious control of psychic life

Nectarine ▲✚ — psycho-spiritual balance

Northern Twayblade ❖ — awareness of spiritual consciousness of nature

Passion Flower ▲▼✚ — spiritual awakening in a balanced integrated way

Patchouli ✚ — spiritual inspiration

Psycho Orchid ✚ — spiritual balance

Purple Monkeyflower ▲ — profound fear of spiritual opening

Queen Anne's Lace ▲▼✚ — integration of sexuality with psychic awareness

Rock Rose ●✚ — identification with higher self when facing threat of death

Rock Water ● — overly strict approach to spiritual life

Rosa Gallica Officinalis ✚ — spiritual rejuvenation

Rosa Horrida ✚ — spiritual sadness

Rosemary ▲▼✚ — feeling ill at ease in physical body

St. John's Wort ▲▼✚ — protection during out-of-body experiences

Shooting Star ▲✚❖ — connection to inner spiritual guidance

Silversword ✚ — spiritual awakening

Star Tulip ▲✚ — receptivity to spiritual worlds

Sweet Chestnut ●✚ — faith when facing the "dark night of the soul"

Washington Lily ✚ — spiritual perseverance

● BACH — ■ MASTER'S — ▲ FES — ▼ GREEN HOPE — ◆ AUSTRALIAN BUSH
❱ LIVING/AUSTRALIA — ❖ ALASKAN — ✚ PEGASUS — ✪ PERELANDRA

White Hibiscus ▼ — increases psychic/sensory abilities to the higher planes of being

White Nymph Water Lily ◗ — uncovering of the deepest spiritual core

Yarrow ▲ — overexpansion of spiritual self leading to acute sensitivity

Spontaneity

Cayenne ▲✚ — fiery catalyst for change

Golden Waitsia ◗ — to re-ignite spontaneity and carefree feelings

Iris ▲ — artistic creativity, inspired approach to the commonplace

Larch ●✚ — flowing creative expression, not censoring self

Plantain ▲ — restores joy and spontaneity

Rock Water ● — flowing attitude toward life, letting go of rigidity

Zinnia ▲▼✚✪ — childlike laughter and delight

Stability

Black-Eyed Susan ▲▼◆ — emotional stability

Chamomile ▲✚ — emotional stability

Chiming Bells ✤ — joy, peace and stability

Chinese Hat Plant ▼ — balance and stability

Clematis ●✚ — memory and emotional stability

Coffee ▲✚ — stabilizes emotions

Green Rose ✚◗ — emotional stability

Many Headed Dryandra ◗ — stability and fulfillment come together at last

Passion Flower ▲▼✚ — stability, eliminates emotional confusion

Potato ✚ — sense of stability in growth process

W.A. Smokebrush ◗ — to reintegrate subtle/physical aspects of being

Strength

Allamanda ✚ — inner strength, inner confidence

Black Cohosh ▲ — confronting and transforming darker psychic energy

Butterfly Lily ✚ — strength of purpose

California Pitcher Plant ▲✚ — courage and strength by harnessing instinctive forces

Centaury ● — courage and strength to say no

Coconut ■ — strong, steady energy

Echinacea ▲✚ — strengthening core integrity

● BACH — ■ MASTER'S — ▲ FES — ▼ GREEN HOPE — ◆ AUSTRALIAN BUSH
◗ LIVING/AUSTRALIA — ✤ ALASKAN — ✚ PEGASUS — ✪ PERELANDRA

Fairy Lantern ▲ — strength to become fully adult

Goddess Grasstree ◗ — metamorphosis to inner strength

Golden Yarrow ▲ — strength and centeredness

Happy Wanderer ◗ — inspiration to stand on own feet

Indian Pink ▲✚ — maintaining inner center of gravity despite intense activity

Lion's Tail ✚ — builds strength and courage

Milkweed ▲✚ — ego strength to cope with core identity

Money Plant ✚ — balance between material and spiritual desires

Mountain Pennyroyal ▲ — strength and clarity of thought

Mountain Pride ▲✚ — courage to take risks, to stand up and speak out

Nicotiana ▲ — false persona of strength or toughness

Oak ●✚ — endurance

Pear ■▲▼✚ — ability to handle crisis

Penstemon ▲✚ — inner strength in the face of adversity

Pink Yarrow ▲ — emotional strength

Red Grevillia ◆ — strength to leave unpleasant situations

Russian Forget-Me-Not ◗ — resilience

Quince ▲✚ — conflict between showing strength and emotional warmth

Scotch Broom ▲✚ — tenacity of purpose in spite of obstacles

Snapdragon ▲▼✚ — strong personal power, often misdirected as aggression

Strawberry ■▲✚ — strong, quiet sense of self and self-worth

Sunflower ▲▼✚❖ — healthy ego strength, strong, radiant individuality

Tomato ■▼✚✪ — the purposeful warrior

Walnut ●✚ — courage to follow one's own path despite outer influences

Yarrow ▲ — integrity of the aura

Yarrow Special Formula ▲ — strengthening mind/body against toxins

Yerba Santa ▲✚ — wasting away of strength

Stress

Aloe Vera ▲▼✚ — overwork, burnout

Bamboo ✚ — alleviates stress

Cacao ✚ — promotes increased mental clarity and reduces stress

Catnip ✚ — releases stress and irrational fear

Cedar ✚ — eases stress

Chamomile ▲✚ — calming and soothing

Cherry Plum ●✚ — fear that extreme stress will lead to breakdown/loss of control

Clove ✚ — eases stress, hypertension, anxiety, headaches, and mental weakness

Coriander ✚ — for poor memory and stress

Corn ■▲▼✚✪ — overwhelmed by city life

Crowea ◆ — worrying, out of balance, feeling "not quite right"

Dahlia ✚ — extreme emotional stress

Dill ▲▼✪ — overstimulation

Elecampagne ✚ — hypochondria and stress

Elm ●✚ — overburdened/overwhelmed by responsibility

Emergency Care Solution ▼ — the Green Hope version of Rescue Remedy

Emergency Essence ◆ — the Australian Bush version of Rescue Remedy

Flax ✚ — emotional stress

Ginseng ✚ — eases stress

Impatiens ●✚ — impatience, frustration, irritation

Indian Pink ▲✚ — overwhelmed by intensity of surrounding activity

Kiwi ✚ — eases stress and moodiness

Labrador Tea ❖ — moving from an unbalanced state to a centered, energized state

Lavender ▲✚ — nervous overwhelm

Lettuce ■✚ — "the unruffler"

Mock Orange ✚ — stress reduction

Okra ✚ — for stress, very grounding

Orchid ✚ — balances emotions in extreme stress

Peanut ✚ — high stress, paranoia

Pecan ✚ — eases self-consciousness of being too tall, short or fat

Pink Yarrow ▲ — emotional negativity from others

Pleurisy Root ✚ — stress and anxiety

Purple Flag Flower ◗ — releasing pressure and tension

Rescue Remedy (Five Flower Formula) ● — overall recovery from stress

Rice ✚ — eases high stress

Rose-Beauty Secret ✚ — eases stress, stimulates balance in city environments

---

● BACH — ■ MASTER'S — ▲ FES — ▼ GREEN HOPE — ◆ AUSTRALIAN BUSH
◗ LIVING/AUSTRALIA — ❖ ALASKAN — ✚ PEGASUS — ✪ PERELANDRA

Rose-Honorine de Brabant ✚ — elimination of stress, hysteria, anxiety
Rosemary ▲▼✚ — feeling cold and depleted under stress
Sandalwood ✚ — fear of heights, insomnia, depression, and stress
Sassafras ✚ — releases stress
Sensitive Plant ✚ — extremely shy and withdrawn or introverted, eases stress
Star of Bethlehem ●▼◗ — soothing severe stress and trauma
Sycamore ✚ — recharges and uplifts when stressed
Valerian ▲✚ — promotes relaxation, contentment
Vervain ●✚ — overenthusiasm/extremism, leading to breakdown or depletion
Yarrow ▲ — stress from negative thoughts/intentions from others
Yarrow Special Formula ▲ — stress from exposure to computers/radiation/etc.
Yellow Flag Flower ◗ — lightheartedness/calmness despite rising tension/pressure

Study

Bedstraw ✚ — inability to study
Chestnut Bud ●✚ — to learn from past mistakes
Cosmos ▲▼✚ — organizing/harmonizing thought processes into coherence
Dandelion ▲▼✚❖ — extreme tension in neck/shoulders from excessive desk work
Hound's Tongue ▲✚ — overly analytical, materialistic thinking
Iris ▲ — artistic and soulful impulses into study
Lavender ▲✚ — nerves depleted from too much study
Madia ▲✚ — concentration and focus
Nasturtium ▲▼✚✪ — over intellectualization, lacking vitality
Peppermint ▲✚ — mental alertness
Pink Trumpet Flower ◗ — harnessing inner strength of purpose, direct it to goals
Purple Enamel Orchid ◗ — consistency in achievement and energy output
Rabbitbrush ▲✚ — mastering many details at one time
Sassafras ✚ — for planning and execution
Shasta Daisy ▲ — integrating information into a whole

W.A. Smokebrush ◗ — difficult concentration, vagueness, feeling muddled

Yarrow Special Formula ▲ — depletion from many hours in front of a computer

Yellow Boronia ◗ — focus and concentration

Yellow Leschenaultia ◗ — calms the mind, helpful with learning disabilities

Zinnia ▲▼✚✪ — too much study, overly serious and somber personality

Surrender

Angel's Trumpet ▲✚ — soul surrender at time of death

Aspen ● — trust in spiritual guidance when facing the unknown

Centaury ● — being a doormat for others

Cherry Plum ●✚ — surrender to the wisdom of the higher self/higher power

Love-Lies-Bleeding ▲ — accepting/enduring physical or emotional pain

Mountain Wormwood ❖ — releasing resentment toward self or others

Oak ●✚ — struggling beyond limits, not knowing when to surrender

Rock Rose ●✚ — surrender/trust when facing death or initiation experience

Sweet Chestnut ●✚ — faith when facing the "dark night of the soul"

Wild Rose ● — apathy/resignation when faced with illness/challenge

Synthesis

Chestnut Bud ●✚ — understanding experiences so they need not be repeated

Cosmos ▲▼✚ — integration of speech with thinking

Cyclamen ✚ — synthesis of information

Daisy ✚ — integrating information into a whole

Lotus ▲✚ — seeing self as expression of spirituality

Rabbitbrush ▲✚ — mastering many details at one time

Shasta Daisy ▲ — integrating information into a whole

Tension

Balsam Poplar ❖ — releasing sexual tension stemming from abuse

California Bay Laurel ✚ — tension in the head and nervous system

---

● BACH — ■ MASTER'S — ▲ FES — ▼ GREEN HOPE — ◆ AUSTRALIAN BUSH
◗ LIVING/AUSTRALIA — ❖ ALASKAN — ✚ PEGASUS — ✪ PERELANDRA

Chamomile ▲✚ — releasing emotional tension held in stomach

Dandelion ▲▼✚❖ — extreme tension in neck/shoulders

Fig ■▲✚ — rigidity, tension, uncompromising nature

Garlic ▲✚ — paralysis in solar plexus due to fear, stage fright

Giant Redwood ▼ — releases tension in pelvic and abdominal muscles

Glastonbury Thorn ▼ — immediate relaxation and release from tension

Golden Yarrow ▲ — tension when performing/speaking due to oversensitivity

Grapefruit ▲▼✚ — releases tension in cranial plates, head, jaw and face

Hyssop ▲▼✚ — releases tension throughout body

Impatiens ●✚ — mental tension and impatience

Iris ▲ — tension in the neck region, unable to feel inner freedom of soul

Lavender ▲✚ — nervous overwhelm

Lilac ▲▼✚ — tension in the back

Nicotiana ▲ — coping with tension by using addictive substances, especially tobacco

Passion Flower ▲▼✚ — tension release

Pear ■▲▼✚ — ability to handle crisis

Petunia ▲✚ — eases tensions, lifts moods

Purple Flag Flower ◗ — releasing pressure and tension

Purple Monkeyflower ▲ — extreme tension or fear, especially of spiritual experiences

Snapdragon ▲▼✚ — holding tension in jaw/mouth, grinding teeth

Soapberry ❖ — release tension from the heart associated with a fear of nature

Spinach ■ — feeling burdened, overwhelmed

Vervain ●✚ — extreme intensity leading to physical tension

Yellow Flag Flower ◗ — lightheartedness/calmness despite rising tension/pressure

Yerba Santa ▲✚ — releasing emotional tension held in the chest region

Ylang Ylang ✚ — calms anger, frustration, stress, depression, insomnia

Thinking

Amaranthus ✚ — clear thinking

Angelica ▲▼✚ — to spiritualize thinking forces

Blackberry ■▲▼✚ — creative power of thought

● BACH — ■ MASTER'S — ▲ FES — ▼ GREEN HOPE — ◆ AUSTRALIAN BUSH
◗ LIVING/AUSTRALIA — ❖ ALASKAN — ✚ PEGASUS — ✪ PERELANDRA

Color Orchid ✚ — creative thinking

Cosmos ▲▼✚ — integration of speech with thinking

Hound's Tongue ▲✚ — overly analytical, materialistic thinking

Impatiens ●✚ — finishing others' thoughts for them

Jacaranda ◆ — decisiveness, clear mindedness, quick thinking

Mountain Pennyroyal ▲ — strength and clarity of thought

Nasturtium ▲▼✚✪ — over intellectualization, lacking vitality

Peppermint ▲✚ — mental alertness

Rabbitbrush ▲✚ — mastering many details at one time

Shasta Daisy ▲ — integrating information into a whole

White Chestnut ● — repetitive and obsessive thoughts

Time Relationship (see Nostalgia)

Tolerance (see Intolerance)

Transcendence

Angel's Trumpet ▲✚ — transcendence of soul from physical plane

Baby Blue Eyes ▲▼ — rebuilding innocence and trust within the soul

Echinacea ▲✚ — reconstellating the self

Grape ■ — loving without condition, demand or expectation

Hound's Tongue ▲✚ — spiritualizing overly materialistic thinking

Iris ▲ — rising above the mundane routine to heightened levels of creativity

Love-Lies-Bleeding ▲ — accepting/enduring physical or emotional pain

Orange ■ — cultivating an inner smile

Rock Rose ●✚ — surrender/trust when facing death or initiation experience

Sagebrush ▲✚ — experiencing inner space within the soul

Sunflower ▲▼✚❖ — raising lower ego to the "sun self"

Sweet Chestnut ●✚ — faith when facing the "dark night of the soul"

Transition

Angel's Trumpet ▲✚ — moving from earthly life to spiritual existence

Cow Parsnip ❖ — contentment during times of transitions

Forget-Me-Not ▲✚❖ — transforming relationship with one who has died

---

● BACH — ■ MASTER'S — ▲ FES — ▼ GREEN HOPE — ◆ AUSTRALIAN BUSH
◗ LIVING/AUSTRALIA — ❖ ALASKAN — ✚ PEGASUS — ✪ PERELANDRA

Hairy Butterwort ✤ — completion of learning cycles without crisis or illness

Morning Glory ▲▼✚ — gaining a fresh perspective

Pale Pink Rose ▼ — eases stress during transitional periods

Poison Ivy ▲✚ — to go from feeling shamed to feeling blessed

Sagebrush ▲✚ — letting go of inessentials no longer serving a purpose

Victoria Regia ✚ — explosive energy, transformation, transition

Walnut ●✚ — breaking free of old ties and habits

Trapped

Cayenne ▲✚ — fiery catalyst for change

Honeysuckle ●✚ — resistance to being in the present

Larch ●✚ — expecting failure, lack of belief in own talents/capacities

Nasturtium ▲▼✚✪ — dysfunctionally absorbing emotional energies of others

Red Grevillia ◆ — strength to leave unpleasant situations

Sunshine Wattle ◆ — stuck in the past

Trauma (see Emergency)

Trust

Angelica ▲▼✚ — deep trust in the divine guidance of our lives

Aspen ● — trust in spiritual guidance when facing the unknown

Baby Blue Eyes ▲▼ — rebuilding innocence and trust within the soul

Basil ▲✚✪ — building trust through communication and openness in relationships

Bog Rosemary ✤ — release of fear through trust

Cerato ●✚ — trusting inner guidance

Cherry Plum ●✚ — surrender to the wisdom of the higher self/higher power

Flannel Flower ◆ — gentleness, sensitivity in touching, joy, trust, sensuality

Forget-Me-Not ▲✚✤ — trusting intuition and inner knowing

Hawthorne ✚ — trust, forgiveness, helps to cleanse the heart of negativity

Mallow ▲▼✚ — learning to trust as a basis of relationships

Mariposa Lily ▲ — trusting bonding relationship between mother and child

---

● BACH — ■ MASTER'S — ▲ FES — ▼ GREEN HOPE — ◆ AUSTRALIAN BUSH
❱ LIVING/AUSTRALIA — ✤ ALASKAN — ✚ PEGASUS — ✪ PERELANDRA

Marjoram ✚ — emotional release, especially fear, leading to trust

Oregon Grape ▲ — trusting the good will of others

Prickly Wild Rose ❖ — allows heart to open in response to conflict

Purple Monkeyflower ▲ — deep trust in spiritual identity and experience

St. John's Wort ▲▼✚ — trust in divine protection

Self-Heal ▲ — trust in own self-healing powers

Spinach ■ — feeling burdened, overwhelmed with mild distrust to paranoia

White Violet ❖ — appropriate boundaries from divine trust

Victim Mentality

Canyon Dudleya ▲ — allowing small episodes to appear overly dramatic

Centaury ● — being a doormat for others

Dogwood ▲ — awkward, accident-prone, feeling unlovable, a victim

Larkspur ▲✚ — excessive dutifulness

Love-Lies-Bleeding ▲ — intense attachment to personal pain and suffering

Southern Cross ◆❱ — personal power, positive attitude, taking responsibility

Urchin Dryandra ❱ — self worth, understanding of how one got into victimhood

Willow ●✚ — seeing self as a victim, blaming others

Violence

Black Cohosh ▲ — abusive, exploitative, incestuous relationships

Dogwood ▲ — self-destructive tendencies

Mountain Devil ◆ — hatred, jealousy, holding grudges, suspicion

Onion ▲✚ — domestic violence/sexual abuse

Orange Spiked Pea ❱ — articulation of feeling without being moved to violence

Scarlet Monkeyflower ▲ — power and anger issues in relationships

Vitality

Aloe Vera ▲▼✚ — reviving exhausted creative forces

Alpine Lily ▲ — more vital female energy when feminine is ungrounded

---

● BACH — ■ MASTER'S — ▲ FES — ▼ GREEN HOPE — ◆ AUSTRALIAN BUSH
❱ LIVING/AUSTRALIA — ❖ ALASKAN — ✚ PEGASUS — ✪ PERELANDRA

Arnica ▲✚ — repairing life energy after shock or trauma

Bignonia ▼ — robust vitality, enthusiasm and joy

California Wild Rose ▲✚ — enthusiasm for life, overcoming apathy

Comfrey ▲▼✚✪ — vitality, tension elimination

Corn ■▲▼✚✪ — grounding spiritual energy through the body

Dill ▲▼✪ — to change perception of being a victim to seeing one's power

Fawn Lily ▲ — vitality which is depleted from overemphasis on spiritual life

Hibiscus ▲ — sexual vitality and responsiveness

Indian Paintbrush ▲✚ — stimulating vitality in creativity

Ixora ▼ — sexual energy, relationship-enhancer for heterosexual couples

Lady's Slipper ▲✤ — nervous exhaustion and sexual depletion

Leafless Orchid ◗ — feelings of depletion for those who work in service to others

Macrocarpa ◆ — renews enthusiasm, vitality

Morning Glory ▲▼✚ — reawakening life energy

Mountain Pennyroyal ▲ — strength and clarity of thought

Nasturtium ▲▼✚✪ — needing more earthly vitality

Orange ■ — energy, renewed interest in life

Peppermint ▲✚ — mental alertness

Pumpkin ▼✚ — physical vitality and commitment

Self-Heal ▲ — awakening self-healing powers

Trumpet Vine ▲✚ — lively creative expression

Wild Rose ● — rallying life forces to fight a long illness

Vulnerability

Angel of Protection ✚ — vulnerability, need of protection

Centaury ● — servile mentality which depletes strength

Golden Yarrow ▲ — extreme sensitivity and vulnerability

Grape ■ — feeling disconnected, alienated, vulnerable

Love-Lies-Bleeding ▲ — easily wounded, or suffering greatly

Monkshood ▲✚✤ — feel vulnerable and have difficulty allowing others true access

Nicotiana ▲ — becoming more vulnerable, more in touch with real feelings

● BACH — ■ MASTER'S — ▲ FES — ▼ GREEN HOPE — ◆ AUSTRALIAN BUSH
◗ LIVING/AUSTRALIA — ✤ ALASKAN — ✚ PEGASUS — ✪ PERELANDRA

Pansy ▲✚ — vulnerable and susceptible

Pear ■▲▼✚ — ability to handle crisis

Pink Monkeyflower ▲ — showing softer, more vulnerable emotions

Pink Yarrow ▲ — susceptibility to emotional influences

Poison Oak ▲ — fear of vulnerability, projecting a hard exterior

Red Clover ▲▼ — susceptibility to group panic and hysteria

Ruta (Rue) ▲✚ — extreme vulnerability to others and to the environment

St. John's Wort ▲▼✚ — extreme vulnerability to psychic influences

Yarrow ▲ — being easily affected by the negative attitudes and intentions of others

Yarrow Special Formula ▲ — susceptibility to negative influences in environment

Warmth

Calendula ▲▼✚ — healing warmth of words

California Wild Rose ▲✚ — igniting the heart

Cayenne ▲✚ — fiery warmth in the will forces

Fawn Lily ▲ — unthawing spiritual forces

Hibiscus ▲ — integration of soul warmth and sexual passion

Mallow ▲▼✚ — creating warmth in contact with others

Mariposa Lily ▲ — feeling surrounded by a mantle of warmth and love

Mesquite ✚ — amplifies compassion and warmth, great for loners

Nasturtium ▲▼✚✪ — thinking forces too cool and detached

Red Hibiscus ▼ — sexual warmth and responsiveness

Rhododendron ✚ — warmth, consolation and a sense of joy

Rosemary ▲▼✚ — feeling cold and depleted under stress

Sticky Monkeyflower ▲ — warmth and intimacy in relationships

Yellow Star Tulip ▲ — warm and compassionate attention for others

Will

Blackberry ■▲▼✚ — putting ideas into action, overcoming inertia

Blue China Orchid ◗ — to strengthen will and take back control of self

Bunchberry ❖ — mental steadfastness and emotional clarity in demanding situations

California Wild Rose ▲✚ — igniting the heart

Cayenne ▲✚ — fiery warmth in the will forces

Centaury ● — courage and strength to say No

Indian Paintbrush ▲✚ — to revive creative expression

Mountain Pride ▲✚ — courage to take risks, to stand up and speak out

Oak ●✚ — endurance

Penstemon ▲✚ — inner strength in the face of adversity

Saguaro ▲✚ — resistance to authority

Snapdragon ▲▼✚ — misplaced forces of will, aggression and verbal abuse

Tansy ▲✚ — resistance to true expression of one's energy

Trillium ▲▼✚ — will forces devoted to survival or materialistic goals

Vervain ●✚ — using personal will to convert others to one's view

Vine ●✚ — darkened forces of the will which control others

Wild Rose ● — rallying life forces to fight a long illness

Wisdom

Black Spruce ✤ — accessing eternal wisdom of nature

California Bay Laurel ✚ — wisdom, flexibility

California Poppy ▲▼ — knowing spiritual wisdom is within

Cerato ●✚ — trusting inner guidance

Chestnut Bud ●✚ — learning lessons of life experience

Cosmos ▲▼✚ — expressing wisdom in speech

Hound's Tongue ▲✚ — spiritualizing thinking process

Lotus ▲✚ — spiritual wisdom

Maltese Cross ▼ — divine wisdom

Mountain Laurel ✚ — conscious understanding and deeper wisdom

Nutmeg ✚ — to draw on wisdom from past lives and one's future life

Pampas Grass ✚ — promotes higher wisdom

Pineapple ■✚ — wisdom, clarity

Pyrola Elliptica ▼ — to bring wisdom of unconscious into focus and understanding

Sage ▲✚ — discovering inner wisdom of life experiences

Saguaro ▲✚ — openness to ancient wisdom, knowledge of elders

Shasta Daisy ▲ — integrating information into a whole

Sitka Spruce Pollen ✤ — integrating wisdom from past experiences

Star Tulip ▲✚ — receptivity to spiritual wisdom through meditation/dreams

White Spruce ✤ — integrating wisdom from past experiences

● BACH — ■ MASTER'S — ▲ FES — ▼ GREEN HOPE — ◆ AUSTRALIAN BUSH
◗ LIVING/AUSTRALIA — ✤ ALASKAN — ✚ PEGASUS — ✪ PERELANDRA

Work and Career Goals

Almond ■▲✚ — workaholism

Bedstraw ✚ — inability to focus on career

Blackberry ■▲▼✚ — putting ideas into action, overcoming inertia

Blue China Orchid ❱ — lack of direction and purpose

Buttercup ▲✚ — accepting the worth of one's life, vocation or lifestyle

California Poppy ▲▼ — inability to settle or commit to a career

California Wild Rose ▲✚ — lack of enthusiasm for one's work

Canyon Dudleya ▲ — inability to accept ordinary
routine/responsibilities

Cayenne ▲✚ — fiery catalyst for change

Centaury ● — overly servile attitude to work

Dandelion ▲▼✚✤ — tendency to overwork

Elm ●✚ — overburdened/overwhelmed by responsibility

Fairy Lantern ▲ — irresponsible work patterns

Fawn Lily ▲ — feeling work is chaotic/stressful, preferring
retreat/isolation

Foxglove ▲✤✚ — fortitude/stamina for long-range and goals and career
plans

Hornbeam ● — "Monday morning blues"

Impatiens ●✚ — feeling impatient when working with others

Iris ▲ — feeling bored with work or career

Lady's Slipper ▲✤ — work which does not reflect real destiny

Larch ●✚ — expecting failure, lack of belief in own talents/capacities

Larkspur ▲✚ — providing leadership with joy, charisma

Nutmeg ✚ — uncertain about career goals

Oak ●✚ — learning how to receive help from others

Pineapple ■✚ — inability to choose a career and stick with it

Pomegranate ▲▼✚ — conflict between family and career

Quaking Grass ▲✚ — difficulty working with group process

Rabbitbrush ▲✚ — mastering many details at one time

Silver Princess ◆ — life purpose and direction, motivation

Tansy ▲✚ — procrastinating, lethargic, overly phlegmatic, indecisive

Trillium ▲▼✚ — desire to work motivated by survival/material
accumulation

Vine ●✚ — compulsion to be in control or dominant when working
with others

● BACH — ■ MASTER'S — ▲ FES — ▼ GREEN HOPE — ◆ AUSTRALIAN BUSH
❱ LIVING/AUSTRALIA — ✤ ALASKAN — ✚ PEGASUS — ✪ PERELANDRA

Wild Oat ● — becoming more serious/directed about life and vocation

Zinnia ▲▼✚✪ — workaholism

Worry

Apple ■▲✚ — worry, doubt, indecision

Brown Boronia ❱ — worried and therefore missing out on joy

Chamomile ▲✚ — calming and soothing

Crowea ◆ — worrying, out of balance, feeling "not quite right"

Feverfew ▲▼ — breaks up deep seated anger, despair, worry, confusion, depression

Filaree ▲✚ — letting go of trivial/petty worries

Garlic ▲✚ — release of nervous fears and insecurities

Golden Waitsia ❱ — to re-ignite spontaneity and carefree feelings

Heather ●✚ — compulsion to talk about problems

Lavender ▲✚ — nervous overwhelm

Red Chestnut ●✚ — obsessive worry and concern about others

Spinach ■ — feeling burdened, overwhelmed with mild distrust to paranoia

Valerian ▲✚ — promotes relaxation, contentment

White Chestnut ● — repetitive and obsessive thoughts

Wild Violet ❱ — fatalism and negativity about life in general

PHYSICAL
SYMPTOMS

Abscess/Boils

Avocado ■▲▼✚
Dagger Hakea ◆
Loofa (Lufa) ▲✚
Mountain Devil ◆
Saguaro ▲✚

Abuse, Accidents, Trauma in Mental/Emotional Section

Aches

Bluebell ◆
Dandelion ▲▼✚❖
Five Corners ◆
Tall Yellow Top ◆

Acidity

Chamomile ▲✚
Jasmine ▲▼✚

Acne

Billy Goat Plum ◆
Five Corners ◆
Loofa (Lufa) ▲✚
Spinifex ◆❭

Addiction in Mental/Emotional Section

Adenoids

Dagger Hakea ◆
Red Helmet Orchid ◆

Adrenals

Almond ■▲✚
Black-Eyed Susan ▲▼◆
Borage ▲▼✚
Chamomile ▲✚

● BACH — ■ MASTER'S — ▲ FES — ▼ GREEN HOPE — ◆ AUSTRALIAN BUSH
❭ LIVING/AUSTRALIA — ❖ ALASKAN — ✚ PEGASUS — ✪ PERELANDRA

Comfrey ▲▼✚✪
Macrocarpa ◆

Aging in Mental/Emotional Section

AIDS

Chaparral ▲✚
Illawara Flame Tree ◆
Lotus ▲✚
Pansy ▲✚
Saguaro ▲✚
Sturt Desert Rose ◆
Waratah ◆

Allergies

Acacia ✚
Apricot ▲✚
Dagger Hakea ◆
Fringed Violet ◆
Goldenrod ▲▼✚
Green Rose ✚❸
Lantana ✚
Snapdragon ▲▼✚
Yarrow ▲
Yarrow Special Formula ▲

Alzheimers

Mallow ▲▼✚

Amenorrhea (see Menstruation — Absence)

Amnesia

Isopogon ◆
Little Flannel Flower ◆
Red Lily ◆
Sundew ◆

Anemia

Bluebell ◆
Five Corners ◆
Kapok Bush ◆
Manzanita ▲✚
Paw Paw ✚◆

Amnesia

Isopogon ◆
Little Flannel Flower ◆

Ankle Problems

Flannel Flower ◆
Isopogon ◆
Sturt Desert Rose ◆

Anorexia Nervosa

Banana ■▲▼✚
Black-Eyed Susan ▲▼◆
Dagger Hakea ◆
Fairy Lantern ▲
Five Corners ◆
Grey Spider Flower ◆
Manzanita ▲✚
Paw Paw ✚◆
Pretty Face ▲

Anus

Bottlebrush ▼◆✚
Sturt Desert Rose ◆

Appendicitis

Apricot ▲✚

Appetite Disorders

Bluebell ◆

● BACH — ■ MASTER'S — ▲ FES — ▼ GREEN HOPE — ◆ AUSTRALIAN BUSH
◗ LIVING/AUSTRALIA — ❖ ALASKAN — ✚ PEGASUS — ✪ PERELANDRA

Crowea ◆
Dog Rose ◆
Fennel ✚
Five Corners ◆
Paw Paw ✚◆

Arm Pain

Paw Paw ✚◆

Arteries

Bluebell ◆

Arteriosclerosis

Amaranthus ✚
Bottlebrush ▼◆✚
Isopogon ◆
Mallow ▲▼✚
Peach ■▲✚
Yellow Cowslip Orchid ◆

Arthritis

Dagger Hakea ◆
Hibbertia ◆
Isopogon ◆
Little Flannel Flower ◆
Mountain Devil ◆
Snapdragon ▲▼✚
Southern Cross ◆❱
Sturt Desert Pea ◆
Yellow Cowslip Orchid ◆
Zinnia ▲▼✚✪

Assimilation (of Nutrients)

Cedar ✚
Jasmine ▲▼✚
Magnolia ▲✚

● BACH — ■ MASTER'S — ▲ FES — ▼ GREEN HOPE — ◆ AUSTRALIAN BUSH
❱ LIVING/AUSTRALIA — ❖ ALASKAN — ✚ PEGASUS — ✪ PERELANDRA

Paw Paw ✚◆
Self-Heal ▲
Star Jasmine ▲

Asthma

Bloodroot ▲▼✚
Bluebell ◆
Daisy ✚
Eucalyptus ▲✚
Green Rose ✚◗
Grey Spider Flower ◆
Hyssop ▲▼✚
Lungwort ✚
Red Grevillia ◆
Tall Mulla Mulla ◆
Tall Yellow Top ◆

Athlete's Foot

Self-Heal ▲

Atonic Dyspepsia

Bloodroot ▲▼✚

Aura — Broken

Fringed Violet ◆

Aura — Misaligned

Crowea ◆

Autolysis

Sage ▲✚

Back/Neck Problems

Banana ■▲▼✚
Centaury ●
Crowea ◆

Dandelion ▲▼✚❖
Graniana Rose ▼
Indian Pipe ✚
Iris ▲
Isopogon ◆
Kangaroo Paw ◆
Lilac ▲▼✚
Paw Paw ✚◆
Sunflower ▲▼✚❖
Sunshine Wattle ◆
Vine ●✚
Waratah ◆

Back — Cervical

Bluebell ◆
Paw Paw ✚◆
Tall Yellow Top ◆

Back — Lumbar-Sacral

Crowea ◆
Southern Cross ◆❱

Back — Thoracic

Bottlebrush ▼◆✚
Crowea ◆
Sturt Desert Rose ◆

Bacterial Infections

Amaranthus ✚
Celery ✪
Jasmine ▲▼✚
Pansy ▲✚
Snapdragon ▲▼✚
Star Tulip ▲✚
Sugar Beet ✚
Zinnia ▲▼✚✪

Baldness (see Hair Loss)

Bedwetting (see Enuresis)

Bell's Palsy

Snapdragon ▲▼✚

Bites, Insects

Mountain Devil ◆

Blisters

Fringed Violet ◆
Spinifex ◆❱

Blood Disorders

Avocado ■▲▼✚
Basil ▲✚✪
Bluebell ◆
Bottlebrush ▼◆✚
Periwinkle ✚
Plantain ▲
Radish ▼✚

Blood Pressure — High

Crowea ◆
Five Corners ◆
Morning Glory ▲▼✚
Mountain Devil ◆
Periwinkle ✚
Vine ●✚

Blood Pressure — Low

Five Corners ◆
Kapok Bush ◆
Southern Cross ◆❱

● BACH — ■ MASTER'S — ▲ FES — ▼ GREEN HOPE — ◆ AUSTRALIAN BUSH
❱ LIVING/AUSTRALIA — ✤ ALASKAN — ✚ PEGASUS — ✪ PERELANDRA

Blood Sugar (Balance)

Apricot ▲✚
Avocado ■▲▼✚
Banana ■▲▼✚
Iris ▲
Jasmine ▲▼✚
Sugar Beet ✚

Body Odor

Billy Goat Plum ◆
Dog Rose ◆
Five Corners ◆

Boils (see Abscess)

Bone Fracture

Fringed Violet ◆
Red Helmet Orchid ◆

Bone Marrow

Five Corners ◆

Bones

Banana ■▲▼✚
Jasmine ▲▼✚

Brain Imbalances

Aloe Vera ▲▼✚
Bush Fuchsia ◆
Comfrey ▲▼✚✪
Dill ▲▼✪
Isopogon ◆
Mugwort ▲✚
Sundew ◆

● BACH — ■ MASTER'S — ▲ FES — ▼ GREEN HOPE — ◆ AUSTRALIAN BUSH
◗ LIVING/AUSTRALIA — ✿ ALASKAN — ✚ PEGASUS — ✪ PERELANDRA

Breasts

Banksia Robur ◆
Bottlebrush ▼◆✚
Philotheca ◆

Breathing Troubles

Daisy ✚
Eucalyptus ▲✚
Five Corners ◆
Green Rose ✚◗
Hyssop ▲▼✚
Lungwort ✚
Rhododendron ✚
Sunshine Wattle ◆
Tall Mulla Mulla ◆
Tall Yellow Top ◆
Yerba Santa ▲✚

Bronchial Conditions

California Pitcher Plant ▲✚
Dagger Hakea ◆
Eucalyptus ▲✚
Hyssop ▲▼✚
Jasmine ▲▼✚
Lungwort ✚
Snapdragon ▲▼✚

Bruising

Five Corners ◆
Flannel Flower ◆

Bubonic Plague

Cedar ✚

Bulimia

Billy Goat Plum ◆

● BACH — ■ MASTER'S — ▲ FES — ▼ GREEN HOPE — ◆ AUSTRALIAN BUSH
◗ LIVING/AUSTRALIA — ❖ ALASKAN — ✚ PEGASUS — ✪ PERELANDRA

Black-Eyed Susan ▲▼◆
Grey Spider Flower ◆
Five Corners ◆
Manzanita ▲✛
Paw Paw ✛◆

Burns

Aloe Vera ▲▼✛
Dagger Hakea ◆
Mountain Devil ◆
Mulla Mulla ◆

Caffeine Problems

Angelica ▲▼✛
Coffee ▲✛
Lotus ▲✛
Nectarine ▲✛
Onion ▲✛
Pansy ▲✛
Pomegranate ▲▼✛
Purple Nightshade ✛
Skullcap ✛

Callouses

Bauhinia ◆
Yellow Cowslip Orchid ◆

Cancer

Almond ■▲✛
Aloe Vera ▲▼✛
Apricot ▲✛
Avocado ■▲▼✛
Bloodroot ▲▼✛
Calendula ▲▼✛
Chaparral ▲✛
Cosmos ▲▼✛

● BACH — ■ MASTER'S — ▲ FES — ▼ GREEN HOPE — ◆ AUSTRALIAN BUSH
◗ LIVING/AUSTRALIA — ✣ ALASKAN — ✛ PEGASUS — ✪ PERELANDRA

Dagger Hakea ◆
Dandelion ▲▼✚✣
Forget-Me-Not ▲✚✣
Hawthorne ✚
Hyssop ▲▼✚
Kapok Bush ◆
Lilac ▲▼✚
Mountain Devil ◆
Papaya ▲▼✚
Peach ■▲✚
Pomegranate ▲▼✚
Red Clover ▲▼
Saguaro ▲✚
Slender Rice Flower ◆
Snapdragon ▲▼✚
Spiderwort ✚
Sturt Desert Pea ◆
Sugar Beet ✚
Sunflower ▲▼✚✣

Candida

Amaranthus ✚
Fig ■▲✚
Kangaroo Paw ◆
Pomegranate ▲▼✚
Spinifex ◆◗

Carpal Tunnel (see Repetitive Stress)

Cataracts

Sunshine Wattle ◆
Waratah ◆

Catarrh

Eucalyptus ▲✚
Flannel Flower ◆

● BACH — ■ MASTER'S — ▲ FES — ▼ GREEN HOPE — ◆ AUSTRALIAN BUSH
◗ LIVING/AUSTRALIA — ✣ ALASKAN — ✚ PEGASUS — ✪ PERELANDRA

Jasmine ▲▼✚
Yerba Santa ▲✚

Cellulite

Billy Goat Plum ◆
Bottlebrush ▼◆✚
Dagger Hakea ◆

Cerebral Palsy

Dill ▲▼✪
Saguaro ▲✚

Cheeks

Sturt Desert Rose ◆

Childbirth

Balsam Poplar ✣
Green Bells of Ireland ▼✣
Grove Sandwort ✣
Hairy Butterwort ✣
Shooting Star ▲✚✣
Star of Bethlehem ●▼◗
Sticky Geranium ✣
Noni ▲
Pear ■▲▼✚
Pomegranate ▲▼✚
Watermelon ▲✚

Chin

Five Corners ◆
Tall Yellow Top ◆

Chlamydia (see Sexual Diseases)

Cholesterol Imbalance

Black-Eyed Susan ▲▼◆

Bluebell ◆
Flannel Flower ◆
Little Flannel Flower ◆

Chronic Disease

Bauhinia ◆
Dog Rose ◆
Kapok Bush ◆
Sunshine Wattle ◆

Circulation Problems

Aloe Vera ▲▼✚
Angelica ▲▼✚
Bottlebrush ▼◆✚
Bleeding Heart ▲✚
Bloodroot ▲▼✚
Bluebell ◆
Chaparral ▲✚
Daffodil ▲▼✚
Fireweed ▲✤✚
Flannel Flower ◆
Morning Glory ▲▼✚
Papaya ▲▼✚
Queen Anne's Lace ▲▼✚
Saguaro ▲✚

Colic

Black-Eyed Susan ▲▼◆
Chamomile ▲✚
Paw Paw ✚◆
Sage ▲✚

Colitis

Bottlebrush ▼◆✚
Dog Rose ◆

● BACH — ■ MASTER'S — ▲ FES — ▼ GREEN HOPE — ◆ AUSTRALIAN BUSH
◗ LIVING/AUSTRALIA — ✤ ALASKAN — ✚ PEGASUS — ✆ PERELANDRA

Colon Spasm

Bamboo +
Cedar +
Green Rose +❙

Coma

Red Lily ◆
Sundew ◆

Common Cold

Black-Eyed Susan ▲▼◆
Eucalyptus ▲+
Jacaranda ◆
Jasmine ▲▼+
Pansy ▲+
Paw Paw +◆
Yerba Santa ▲+

Conjunctivitis

Mountain Devil ◆
Sunshine Wattle ◆

Constipation

Bluebell ◆
Bottlebrush ▼◆+ and Boronia ◆
Cedar +
Pomegranate ▲▼+
Tomato ■▼+✪

Convalescence/Recuperation

Golden Waitsia ❙
Hornbeam ●
Lotus ▲+
Pink Fountain Trigger Plant ❙
Self-Heal ▲

Valerian ▲✚
Zucchini ▲▼✚❂

Corns

Bauhinia ◆   .
Isopogon ◆

Coughs

Dagger Hakea ◆
Illawara Flame Tree ◆
Red Helmet Orchid ◆

Cramps

Bottlebrush ▼◆✚
Dampiera ◗
Dandelion ▲▼✚✿
Grey Spider Flower ◆
Impatiens ●✚

Cranial Inflammation

Aloe Vera ▲▼✚

Cuts

Spinifex ◆◗
Sturt Desert Rose ◆

Cystic Fibrosis

Southern Cross ◆◗

Cystitis

Dagger Hakea ◆
Mountain Devil ◆
Pomegranate ▲▼✚
Spinifex ◆◗

Cysts

Mountain Devil ◆
Pomegranate ▲▼✚
Sturt Desert Rose ◆

Deafness

Illawara Flame Tree ◆
Isopogon ◆
Tall Yellow Top ◆

Dehydration

She Oak ◆

Detoxification

Arnica ▲✚
Avocado ■▲▼✚
Bottlebrush ▼◆✚
Chaparral ▲✚
Coffee ▲✚
Coralroot-Spotted ✚
Dandelion ▲▼✚✤
Morning Glory ▲▼✚
Noni ▲
Pine Drops ✚
Skullcap ✚
Sourgrass ✚
Spruce ▲✚

Diabetes (see Hypoglycemia/Diabetes)

Diarrhea

Black-Eyed Susan ▲▼◆
Cedar ✚
Paw Paw ✚◆

Digestive Problems

Aloe Vera ▲▼✚
California Pitcher Plant ▲✚
Cedar ✚
Chamomile ▲✚
Crowea ◆
Dill ▲▼✪
Jasmine ▲▼✚
Red Spider Lily ✚
Sage ▲✚

Dizziness/Faintness/Vertigo

Aspen ●
Bush Fuchsia ◆
Chinese Hat Plant ▼
Clematis ●✚
Jacaranda ◆
W.A. Smokebrush ◗

Dwarfism

Almond ■▲✚
Mango ✚
Yellow Cowslip Orchid ◆

Dysentery

Bloodroot ▲▼✚

Dyslexia

Bush Fuchsia ◆
Jacaranda ◆
Sundew ◆

Ear Problems

Bush Gardenia ◆
Kangaroo Paw ◆
Star Tulip ▲✚
Viburnum ✚

● BACH — ■ MASTER'S — ▲ FES — ▼ GREEN HOPE — ◆ AUSTRALIAN BUSH
◗ LIVING/AUSTRALIA — ✣ ALASKAN — ✚ PEGASUS — ✪ PERELANDRA

Eczema

Aloe Vera ▲▼✚
Apricot ▲✚
Billy Goat Plum ◆
Bloodroot ▲▼✚
Dagger Hakea ◆
Loofa (Lufa) ▲✚
Saguaro ▲✚
Spinifex ◆❱

Elbow

Bauhinia ◆
Bottlebrush ▼◆✚

Elimination

Avocado ■▲▼✚
Cedar ✚
Chamomile ▲✚
Star Jasmine ▲

Endocrine System

Lotus ▲✚

Energy, Environmental Cleansing in Mental/Emotional Section

Enuresis

Dog Rose ◆
Red Helmet Orchid ◆

Epilepsy

Angelica ▲▼✚
Green Rose ✚❱

Epistaxis

Illawara Flame Tree ◆

● BACH — ■ MASTER'S — ▲ FES — ▼ GREEN HOPE — ◆ AUSTRALIAN BUSH
❱ LIVING/AUSTRALIA — ❖ ALASKAN — ✚ PEGASUS — ✪ PERELANDRA

Epstein Barr Virus

Banksia Robur ◆
Bottlebrush ▼◆✚
Cosmos ▲▼✚
Date Palm ▼✚
Five Corners ◆
Lettuce ■✚
Macrocarpa ◆
Pansy ▲✚

Exhaustion in Mental/Emotional Section

Eye Problems

Alder ✜
Bush Fuchsia ◆
Cotton ▲▼✚
Iris ▲
Nasturtium ▲▼✚✪
Queen Anne's Lace ▲▼✚
Star Tulip ▲✚
Sunshine Wattle ◆

Eyebrows

Dagger Hakea ◆
Mountain Devil ◆

Fallopian Tubes

She Oak ◆
Spinifex ◆❱

Fatigue in Mental/Emotional Section

Fertility

Blackberry ■▲▼✚
Fig ■▲✚
Gooseberry ✚

● BACH — ■ MASTER'S — ▲ FES — ▼ GREEN HOPE — ◆ AUSTRALIAN BUSH
❱ LIVING/AUSTRALIA — ✜ ALASKAN — ✚ PEGASUS — ✪ PERELANDRA

Lady's Mantle ✚
Noni ▲
Pomegranate ▲▼✚
She Oak ◆
Watermelon ▲✚

Fever

Dandelion ▲▼✚❖
Ginseng ✚
Mountain Devil ◆
Mulla Mulla ◆
Onion ▲✚

Finger Pain

Kapok Bush ◆
Sundew ◆

Fluid Retention

California Pitcher Plant ▲✚
She Oak ◆

Food Poisoning

Crowea ◆
Paw Paw ✚◆

Foot Problems

Bauhinia ◆
Bottlebrush ▼◆✚
Dog Rose ◆
Silver Princess ◆
Sunshine Wattle ◆

Forehead

Boronia ◆
Crowea ◆
Paw Paw ✚◆

● BACH — ■ MASTER'S — ▲ FES — ▼ GREEN HOPE — ◆ AUSTRALIAN BUSH
◗ LIVING/AUSTRALIA — ❖ ALASKAN — ✚ PEGASUS — ✪ PERELANDRA

Frigidity

Billy Goat Plum ◆
Flannel Flower ◆
Hibiscus ▲
Ixora ▼
Pumpkin ▼✚
Red Helmet Orchid ◆
Wisteria ◆

Gall Stones

Apricot ▲✚
Dagger Hakea ◆
Slender Rice Flower ◆
Southern Cross ◆❱

Gout

Black-Eyed Susan ▲▼◆
Mountain Devil ◆

Gum Problems

Jacaranda ◆
Peach Flowered Tea Tree ◆

Hair Loss/Baldness

Cedar ✚
Cotton ▲▼✚
Dog Rose ◆
Hibbertia ◆
Lemon ▲▼✚
Yellow Cowslip Orchid ◆

Halitosis (Bad Breath)

Crowea ◆
Mountain Devil ◆
Paw Paw ✚◆

Hay Fever

Eucalyptus ▲✚
Green Rose ✚◗

Headache

Apricot ▲✚
Aspen ●
Black-Eyed Susan ▲▼◆
Clove ✚
Crown of Thorns ✚
Feverfew ▲▼
Five Corners ◆
Grapefruit ▲▼✚
Green Rose ✚◗
Lavender ▲✚
Paw Paw ✚◆
Plantain ▲
Sturt Desert Rose ◆
Vervain ●✚
White Chestnut ●

Heart Problems

Black-Eyed Susan ▲▼◆
Bleeding Heart ▲✚
Bloodroot ▲▼✚
Bluebell ◆
Borage ▲▼✚
Cosmos ▲▼✚
Foxglove ▲✤✚
Hawthorne ✚
Little Flannel Flower ◆
Mallow ▲▼✚
Monkshood ▲✚✤
Old Man Banksia ◆
Peach ■▲✚
Red Helmet Orchid ◆
Rosemary ▲▼✚

Hemorrhoids

Black-Eyed Susan ▲▼◆
Bottlebrush ▼◆✚
Mallow ▲▼✚
Mountain Devil ◆

Herpes (see Sexual Diseases)

Hiccoughs

Black-Eyed Susan ▲▼◆
Crowea ◆
Daisy ✚
Paw Paw ✚◆

Hip Problems

Dog Rose ◆
Old Man Banksia ◆
Sundew ◆
Sunshine Wattle ◆

Hives

Dagger Hakea ◆
Dog Rose ◆
Fringed Violet ◆

Hormone Imbalance — Female

Evening Primrose ▲
Pomegranate ▲▼✚
She Oak ◆
Watermelon ▲✚

Hormone Imbalance — Male

Evening Primrose ▲
Watermelon ▲✚

Hypoglycemia/Diabetes

Date ■

Hyperactivity in Mental/Emotional Section

Immune System

Amaranthus ✚
Apple ■▲✚
Celery ✪
Echinacea ▲✚
Garlic ▲✚
Gorse ●✚
Hawthorne ✚
Lavender ▲✚
Love-Lies-Bleeding ▲
Macrocarpa ◆
Mock Orange ✚
Morning Glory ▲▼✚
Pansy ▲✚

Impotency

Banana ■▲▼✚
Ixora ▼
Larch ●✚

Incontinence

Cedar ✚
St. John's Wort ▲▼✚

Indigestion (Dyspepsia)

Chamomile ▲✚
Sage ▲✚

Inflammation

Apricot ▲✚
Dill ▲▼✪

● BACH — ■ MASTER'S — ▲ FES — ▼ GREEN HOPE — ◆ AUSTRALIAN BUSH
◗ LIVING/AUSTRALIA — ✿ ALASKAN — ✚ PEGASUS — ✪ PERELANDRA

Eucalyptus ▲✚
French Marigold ▼
Garlic ▲✚
Saguaro ▲✚

Influenza

Eucalyptus ▲✚
Jasmine ▲▼✚
Pansy ▲✚

Injury (see *Emergency* in Mental/Emotional Section)

Insomnia in Mental/Emotional Section

Itching

Loofa (Lufa) ▲✚

Jaundice

Eucalyptus ▲✚

Jet Lag

Banksia Robur ◆
Dill ▲▼✪
Lotus ▲✚
Pennyroyal ✚
Sage ▲✚
Ylang Ylang ✚

Kidney Problems

Avocado ■▲▼✚
Bottlebrush ▼◆✚
Chamomile ▲✚
Eucalyptus ▲✚
Kidney Bean ✚
Red Spider Lily ✚
Rice ✚

Laryngitis

Lungwort ✚
Snapdragon ▲▼✚

Liver Problems

Avocado ■▲▼✚
Plantain ▲

Long-Term Illness

Coralroot-Spotted ✚

Lung Imbalance

Eucalyptus ▲✚
Hyssop ▲▼✚
Jasmine ▲▼✚
Lungwort ✚
Manzanita ▲✚
Yerba Santa ▲✚

Lymphatic System

Apricot ▲✚
Avocado ■▲▼✚
Saguaro ▲✚

Malaria

Eucalyptus ▲✚

Massage in Mental/Emotional Section

Meniere's Disease

Green Rose ✚◗

Menopause (also see in Mental/Emotional Section)

Alpine Lily ▲
Borage ▲▼✚
Easter Lily ▲✚

● BACH — ■ MASTER'S — ▲ FES — ▼ GREEN HOPE — ◆ AUSTRALIAN BUSH
◗ LIVING/AUSTRALIA — ❖ ALASKAN — ✚ PEGASUS — ✪ PERELANDRA

Evening Primrose ▲
Fuchsia ▲
Gooseberry ✚
Hibiscus ▲
Impatiens ●✚
Mallow ▲▼✚
Mariposa Lily ▲
Pokeweed ✚
Pomegranate ▲▼✚
Rosemary ▲▼✚
She Oak ◆
Shrimp Plant ✚
Tiger Lily ▲✚

Menstruation — Absence

Evening Primrose ▲
Fairy Lantern ▲
Five Corners ◆
Mugwort ▲✚
Pomegranate ▲▼✚
She Oak ◆

Menstruation — Irregular

Evening Primrose ▲
Fairy Lantern ▲
Mugwort ▲✚
Pomegranate ▲▼✚

Menstruation — Pains

Black Cohosh ▲
Feverfew ▲▼
Love-Lies-Bleeding ▲
Pomegranate ▲▼✚

Metabolism (Re-Balancing)

Jacob's Ladder ✢✚

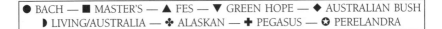

● BACH — ■ MASTER'S — ▲ FES — ▼ GREEN HOPE — ◆ AUSTRALIAN BUSH
◗ LIVING/AUSTRALIA — ✢ ALASKAN — ✚ PEGASUS — ✺ PERELANDRA

Nasturtium ▲▼✚✪
Peppermint ▲✚
Rosemary ▲▼✚
Snapdragon ▲▼✚

Miasms — General

Lotus ▲✚

Miasms — Heavy Metals

Bloodroot ▲▼✚
Daffodil ▲▼✚
Hyssop ▲▼✚

Miasms — Petrochemical

Almond ■▲✚
Apricot ▲✚
Coffee ▲✚

Miasms — Psora

Camphor ✚
Dandelion ▲▼✚❖
Eucalyptus ▲✚
Fig ■▲✚
Garlic ▲✚
Grapefruit ▲▼✚
Lemon ▲▼✚

Miasms — Radiation

Bloodroot ▲▼✚
Garlic ▲✚
Lemon ▲▼✚

Miasms — Syphilitic

Banana ■▲▼✚
Bells of Ireland ▼✚
Bottlebrush ▼◆✚

● BACH — ■ MASTER'S — ▲ FES — ▼ GREEN HOPE — ◆ AUSTRALIAN BUSH
◗ LIVING/AUSTRALIA — ❖ ALASKAN — ✚ PEGASUS — ✪ PERELANDRA

California Poppy ▲▼
Celandine ✚
Chamomile ▲✚
Chaparral ▲✚
Comfrey ▲▼✚✪
Four Leaf Clover ✚
Iris ▲
Jasmine ▲▼✚

Miasms — Sycosis
Dandelion ▲▼✚❖
Lilac ▲▼✚

Miasms — Tuberculosis
Blackberry ■▲▼✚
Cotton ▲▼✚
Eucalyptus ▲✚
Green Rose ✚❱
Hops ✚
Live Forever ✚
Red Clover ▲▼

Migraine
Crown of Thorns ✚
Feverfew ▲▼
Green Rose ✚❱
Plantain ▲

Mosquito Bites
Garlic ▲✚
Mountain Devil ◆

Motion Sickness (see Travel Sickness)

Multiple Sclerosis
California Poppy ▲▼

Comfrey ▲▼✦○
Dandelion ▲▼✦❖

Muscular Disorders

Apricot ▲✦
Bottlebrush ▼◆✦
Comfrey ▲▼✦○
Dandelion ▲▼✦❖
French Marigold ▼
Petunia ▲✦
Vervain ●✦

Nails

Fringed Violet ◆

Nasal Congestion

Eucalyptus ▲✦
Jasmine ▲▼✦
California Pitcher Plant ▲✦
Yerba Santa ▲✦

Nasal-Runny (see Catarrh)

Nausea

Dog Rose ◆
Paw Paw ✦◆
Sage ▲✦

Neck (see Back/Neck Problems)

Nervousness in Mental/Emotional Section

Nervous System (Tonic)

Aloe Vera ▲▼✦
Angelica ▲▼✦
Arnica ▲✦

California Bay Laurel ✚
California Poppy ▲▼
Chamomile ▲✚
Coffee ▲✚
Comfrey ▲▼✚✺
Dill ▲▼✺
Four Leaf Clover ✚
Hawthorne ✚
Hyssop ▲▼✚
Lavender ▲✚
Morning Glory ▲▼✚
Nasturtium ▲▼✚✺
Pear ■▲▼✚
Petunia ▲✚
Skullcap ✚
Sugar Beet ✚
Valerian ▲✚
Viburnum ✚

Neuralgia

Flannel Flower ◆
Sturt Desert Rose ◆

Nosebleed (see Epistaxis)

Obesity

Apricot ▲✚
Banana ■▲▼✚
Evening Primrose ▲
Goldenrod ▲▼✚
Hound's Tongue ▲✚
Nicotiana ▲
Pink Monkeyflower ▲
Tansy ▲✚

Ovaries

She Oak ◆
Turkey Bush ◆

Pain

Cotton Grass ❖
Dog Rose of the Wild Forces ◆
Foxglove ▲❖✚
Illyarrie ◗
Love-Lies-Bleeding ▲
Menzies Banksia ◗
Papaya ▲▼✚
Sturt Desert Rose ◆
Valerian ▲✚

Pancreas

French Marigold ▼
Peach Flowered Tea Tree ◆

Paralysis

Grey Spider Flower ◆
Wild Potato Bush ◆

Parasites

Billy Goat Plum ◆
Five Corners ◆
Flee Free ▼
Garlic ▲✚
Kapok Bush ◆
Southern Cross ◆◗

Pelvic Inflammatory Disease

Billy Goat Plum ◆
Pomegranate ▲▼✚
Spinifex ◆◗

Pineal Gland

Bush Fuchsia ◆

Pituitary Gland

Yellow Cowslip Orchid ◆

PMS

Crowea ◆
Evening Primrose ▲
Feverfew ▲▼
Onion ▲✚
Peach Flowered Tea Tree ◆
Pomegranate ▲▼✚
She Oak ◆

Pregnancy in Mental/Emotional Section

Prostate

Flannel Flower ◆
Kapok Bush ◆
Sturt Desert Rose ◆

Psoriasis

Aloe Vera ▲▼✚
Angelica ▲▼✚
Billy Goat Plum ◆
Little Flannel Flower ◆
Loofa (Lufa) ▲✚
Spinifex ◆❱

Puberty (see *Adolescence*) in Mental/Emotional Section

Radiation Problems

Almond ■▲✚
Bush Fuchsia ◆ plus *Crowea* ◆ plus *Fringed Violet* ◆ plus *Mulla Mulla* ◆ plus *Paw Paw* ✚◆ plus *Waratah* ◆
Eucalyptus ▲✚

● BACH — ■ MASTER'S — ▲ FES — ▼ GREEN HOPE — ◆ AUSTRALIAN BUSH
❱ LIVING/AUSTRALIA — ✤ ALASKAN — ✚ PEGASUS — ✪ PERELANDRA

Spiderwort ✚
Sugar Beet ✚
Yarrow Special Formula ▲

Repetitive Stress Injury
Red Grevillia ◆
Southern Cross ◆◗

Rheumatism
Dagger Hakea ◆
Isopogon ◆
Southern Cross ◆◗
Yellow Cowslip Orchid ◆

Rheumatoid Arthritis
Dagger Hakea ◆
Hibbertia ◆
Red Helmet Orchid ◆
Southern Cross ◆◗
Sturt Desert Pea ◆

Round Shoulders
Dog Rose ◆
Five Corners ◆
Sunshine Wattle ◆
Waratah ◆

Scar Tissue
Aloe Vera ▲▼✚

Sciatica
Crowea ◆
Dog Rose ◆

Senility
Isopogon ◆

● BACH — ■ MASTER'S — ▲ FES — ▼ GREEN HOPE — ◆ AUSTRALIAN BUSH
◗ LIVING/AUSTRALIA — ✣ ALASKAN — ✚ PEGASUS — ✪ PERELANDRA

Red Lily ◆
Sundew ◆

Sexual Diseases (Chlamydia, Herpes) (see also Venereal Disease)

Billy Goat Plum ◆
Pansy ▲✚
Pomegranate ▲▼✚
Spinifex ◆▶
Sturt Desert Rose ◆

Shock in Mental/Emotional Section

Shoulders

Dog Rose ◆
Paw Paw ✚◆
Sunshine Wattle ◆

Sight (Enhancing)

Cotton ▲▼✚
Queen Anne's Lace ▲▼✚

Sickle Cell Anemia

Angelica ▲▼✚

Sinus

Dagger Hakea ◆
Eucalyptus ▲✚
Goldenrod ▲▼✚
Jasmine ▲▼✚

Skin Problems

Aloe Vera ▲▼✚
Angelica ▲▼✚
Billy Goat Plum ◆
Bloodroot ▲▼✚
Bottlebrush ▼◆✚

Eucalyptus ▲✛
Fig ■▲✛
Five Corners ◆
Fringed Violet ◆
Ginseng ✛
Jacaranda ◆
Jasmine ▲▼✛
Loofa (Lufa) ▲✛
Manzanita ▲✛
Red Spider Lily ✛
Spinifex ◆◗

Smoking (Difficulty Quitting)

Boronia ◆ plus Bottlebrush ▼◆✛

Snoring

Isopogon ◆
Old Man Banksia ◆

Speech Problems/Stuttering

Bush Fuchsia ◆
Dog Rose ◆
Five Corners ◆
Larch ●✛
Mimulus ●✛
Petunia ▲✛
Snapdragon ▲▼✛

Spleen

Boronia ◆
Dagger Hakea ◆
Hibbertia ◆

Stiffness

Bauhinia ◆
Hibbertia ◆

● BACH — ■ MASTER'S — ▲ FES — ▼ GREEN HOPE — ◆ AUSTRALIAN BUSH
◗ LIVING/AUSTRALIA — ❖ ALASKAN — ✛ PEGASUS — ✪ PERELANDRA

Isopogon ◆
Little Flannel Flower ◆
Yellow Cowslip Orchid ◆

Stomach Problems
Billy Goat Plum ◆
Crowea ◆
Dog Rose ◆
Paw Paw ✚◆

Stroke
Bauhinia ◆
Black-Eyed Susan ▲▼◆
Kapok Bush ◆
Old Man Banksia ◆
Tall Yellow Top ◆

Sunburn (see Burns)

Swelling (see Inflammation)

Teeth
Banana ■▲▼✚
Jacaranda ◆
Paw Paw ✚◆
Sundew ◆

Teeth — Grinding
Banana ■▲▼✚
Black-Eyed Susan ▲▼◆
Morning Glory ▲▼✚

Testicle Issues
Flannel Flower ◆
She Oak ◆

● BACH — ■ MASTER'S — ▲ FES — ▼ GREEN HOPE — ◆ AUSTRALIAN BUSH
◗ LIVING/AUSTRALIA — ✤ ALASKAN — ✚ PEGASUS — ✪ PERELANDRA

Testosterone Imbalances

Papaya ▲▼✚

Tetanus

Four Leaf Clover ✚

Throat

Bush Fuchsia ◆
Bush Iris ◆
Flannel Flower ◆
Four Leaf Clover ✚
Lungwort ✚
Pansy ▲✚
Pennyroyal ✚
Snapdragon ▲▼✚

Thymus Disorders

Illawara Flame Tree ◆
Jacob's Ladder ✿✚
Southern Cross ◆◗

Thyroid Imbalance

Old Man Banksia ◆
Southern Cross ◆◗
Thyme ▲▼✚

Tonsillitis

Dill ▲▼✪
Jasmine ▲▼✚
Lungwort ✚
Pennyroyal ✚
Snapdragon ▲▼✚

Travel Sickness

Dill ▲▼✪
Dog Rose ◆

● BACH — ■ MASTER'S — ▲ FES — ▼ GREEN HOPE — ◆ AUSTRALIAN BUSH
◗ LIVING/AUSTRALIA — ✿ ALASKAN — ✚ PEGASUS — ✪ PERELANDRA

Fig ■▲✚
Red Grevillia ◆
Ylang Ylang ✚

Ulcer (Peptic)

Cedar ✚
Crowea ◆
Green Rose ✚❱
Monkshood ▲✚❖
Peppermint ▲✚
Pleurisy Root ✚

Urinary Tract Infections (see Cystitis)

Uterus Issues

She Oak ◆
Turkey Bush ◆

Vaginitis

Billy Goat Plum ◆
Dagger Hakea ◆
Sturt Desert Rose ◆

Varicose Veins

Banksia Robur ◆
Paw Paw ✚◆
Red Grevillia ◆

Venereal Disease

Billy Goat Plum ◆
Dagger Hakea ◆
Sturt Desert Rose ◆

Vision (see Sight)

Vomiting

Bauhinia ◆
Paw Paw ✚◆

Warts

Billy Goat Plum ◆
Five Corners ◆
Pansy ▲✚

Weight Control

Dayflower ✚
Dog Rose ◆
Fringed Violet ◆
Hound's Tongue ▲✚
Mango ✚
Mulla Mulla ◆
Old Man Banksia ◆
Wild Potato Bush ◆
Yerba Santa ▲✚

Bibliography

Arnos, Kathy. *Bach Flowers For Children*. New York: Discount Newsletter Printing, 1992

Bach, Edward. *Heal Thyself*. London: CW Daniel Company, 1931 (Appearing in compilation:*The Bach Flower Remedies*. New Canaan, CT: Keats Publishing, 1977, 1979)

_____. *The Twelve Healers*. London: CW Daniel Company, 1933 (Appearing in compilation:*The Bach Flower Remedies*. New Canaan, CT: Keats Publishing, 1977, 1979)

Devi, Lila. *The Essential Flower Essence Handbook*. Canada: Best Book Manufacturers, 1996

Gurudas. *Flower Essences and Vibrational Healing*. San Rafael, CA: Cassandra Press, 1989. No City Listed: Brotherhood of Life, 1983

Harvey, Clare G. and Cochrane, Amanda. *The Encyclopaedia of Flower Remedies*. San Francsico: Thorsons, 1995

Hasnas, Rachelle. *Pocket Guide to Bach Flower Essences*. Freedom, CA: Crossing Press, 1997

Johnson, Steve. *The Essence of Healing: A Guide to the Alaskan Flower, Gem and Enviornmental Essences*. Homer, Alaska: Alaskan Flower Essence Project, 1996

_____. *Flower Essences of Alaska*. Homer, Alaska: Alaskan Flower Essence Project, 1992

Kaminski, Patricia and Katz, Richard. *Flower Essence Repertory: A Comprehensive Guide to North American and English Flower Essences for Emotional and Spiritual Well-Being*. Nevada City, CA: Flower Essence Society, 1986, 1987, 1992, 1994, 1996

Krämer, Dietmar. *New Bach Flower Therapies: Healing the Emotional Causes of Illness*. Rochester, VT: Healing Arts Press, 1995. Interlaken, Switzerland: Ansata-Verlag, 1989.

Mason, Gary, Editor. *The Flower Essence Pharmacy Catalog 1997, Volumes I & II*. Little River, CA: The Flower Essence Pharmacy, 1997

Scheffer, Mechthild. *Bach Flower Therapy: Theory and Practice*. Rochester, VT: Healing Arts Press, 1988. Munich: Heinrich Hugendubel Verlag, 1981.

Sheehan, Molly. *A Guide to Green Hope Farm Flower Essences*. Meriden, NH: Green Hope Farm, 1997

Vlamis, Gregory. *Bach Flower Remedies to the Rescue*. Rochester, VT: Healing Arts Press, 1986, 1988, 1990

Wheeler, F. J. *The Bach Remedies Repertory.* London: CW Daniel Company, 1952 (Appearing in compilation:*The Bach Flower Remedies.* New Canaan, CT: Keats Publishing, 1977, 1979)

White, Ian. *Australian Bush Flower Essences.* Findhorn, Scotland: Findhorn Press, 1993. Australia: Bantam Books(Transworld), 1991.

How to Reach the Makers
of the Flower Remedies

Alaskan Flower Essence Project
PO Box 1369
Homer, Alaska 99603-1369
Phone: (907) 235-2188 / Fax: (907) 235-2777

Australian Bush Flower Essences
8A Oaks Avenue
Dee Why, NSW 2099, Australia
Phone: (2) 9972-1033 / Fax: (2) 9972-1102

Nelson Bach USA Ltd. (Bach Flower Remedies)
1007 West Upsal Street
Philadelphia, PA 19119
Phone: (800) 314-BACH / Fax: (215) 844-6165

Flower Essence Society (Healing Herbs)
(North American and English Essences)
PO Box 459
Nevada City, CA 95959
Phone: (800) 548-0075 / Fax: (916) 265-6467

Green Hope Farm
PO Box 125
True Road
Meriden, NH 03770
Phone: (603) 469-3662

Living Essences of Australia
PO Box 355
Scarborough 6019
Perth, West Australia, Australia
Phone: (9) 443-5600 / Fax: (9) 443-5610

Master's Flower Essences

14618 Tyler-Foote Road
Nevada City, CA 95959
Phone: (800) 347-3639

Pegasus Products

PO Box 228
Boulder, CO 80306
Phone: (800) 527-6104 / Fax: (970) 667-3624

Perelandra

PO Box 3603
Warrenton, VA 22186
Phone: (540) 937-2153 / Fax: (540) 937-3360